ASYMPTOMATIC

ASYMPTOMATIC

The Silent Spread of COVID-19 and the
Future of Pandemics

JOSHUA S. WEITZ

 JOHNS HOPKINS UNIVERSITY PRESS | *Baltimore*

Johns Hopkins University Press
2715 North Charles Street
Baltimore, Maryland 21218
www.press.jhu.edu

Library of Congress Cataloging-in-Publication Data

Names: Weitz, Joshua S., 1975– author.
Title: Asymptomatic : the silent spread of covid-19 and the future of
    pandemics / Joshua S. Weitz.
Description: Baltimore : Johns Hopkins University Press, 2024. | Includes
    bibliographical references and index.
Identifiers: LCCN 2024013758 | ISBN 9781421450483 (paperback) |
    ISBN 9781421450490 (ebook)
Subjects: MESH: Asymptomatic Infections | Basic Reproduction Number |
    COVID-19—epidemiology | COVID-19—transmission | Pandemics |
    SARS-CoV-2
Classification: LCC RA644.C67 | DDC 614.5/924144—dc23/eng/20240408
LC record available at https://lccn.loc.gov/2024013758

A catalog record for this book is available from the British Library.

*Special discounts are available for bulk purchases of this book. For more information,
please contact Special Sales at specialsales@jh.edu.*

Here also I ought to leave a farther Remark for the use of Posterity, concerning the Manner of Peoples infecting one another; namely, that it was not the sick People only, from whom the Plague was immediately receiv'd by others that were sound, but THE WELL. . . .

These were the dangerous People, these were the People of whom the well People ought to have been afraid; but then on the other Side it was impossible to know them.

Daniel Defoe,
A JOURNAL OF THE PLAGUE YEAR (1722)

CONTENTS

Asymptomatic.

The word may seem an unlikely start for a book meant to explain the spread of a disease that has killed more than 1 million Americans and more than 7 million individuals worldwide.

Yet, over time, we have learned that nearly everyone who was infected with SARS-CoV-2 (severe acute respiratory syndrome coronavirus 2) survived—roughly 99% (or more). Not only did the vast majority survive, but many—if not half of those infected—had such mild infections that they never knew they had the virus. They were asymptomatic.

It is precisely because infection with SARS-CoV-2, which causes the disease named COVID-19, so often manifests itself with mild symptoms, the absence of recognizable symptoms, or no symptoms at all that the pandemic has been so hard to control. On the one hand, the existence of asymptomatic infections may suggest that SARS-CoV-2 should not lead to a severe outbreak. But individuals who are asymptomatic can nonetheless transmit an infection to others. And because they are asymptomatic, they are less likely to be aware that they are infected, less likely to take protective measures, and more likely to interact with more people while infectious. The fact that asymptomatically infected individuals can and do infect others is the very mechanism that has allowed SARS-CoV-2 to have such devastating global effects.

We have known since early 2020 that individuals with mild or asymptomatic cases could transmit their infection to others. Scientists and public health experts tried to warn of the risk of the asymptomatic route of transmission—to urge government officials, health care providers, and political decision makers to take action; to caution against the misinterpretation of individual versus population-level outcomes; and to develop appropriate mitigation strategies.

We failed.

We failed because being asymptomatic is a double-edged sword. For COVID-19 skeptics and minimizers, the commonplace nature of asymptomatic infections has been misappropriated as evidence to support claims that the pandemic is a hoax, that there is fundamentally nothing to worry about, and that COVID-19, in effect, is no worse than seasonal flu. For those who have argued that "we're all going to die," the evidence of asymptomatic infections makes for an unassailable counterpoint to worst-case scenarios, which have become even more misaligned with evidence of milder disease outcomes in children and young adults.

The reality is that asymptomatic transmission has profound consequences. Individuals infected with SARS-CoV-2 are nearly as likely to have a mild or asymptomatic infection as they are to have a symptomatic infection. This volatile mix of good and bad outcomes at the individual scale can fuel explosive growth at population scales—a fact that remains poorly understood and too often neglected in the prioritization of public health communication and response to the pandemic.

I began writing this book in early 2022—two years after redirecting my research group's efforts to respond to what was then a novel coronavirus spreading in the Wuhan Province of China. Since January 2020, our Quantitative Viral Dynamics group has worked collaboratively with scientists in the United States and worldwide to estimate COVID-19's potential strength and severity, to implement mitigation programs (including large-scale viral testing at Georgia Tech that delivered more than 500,000 free tests to help protect the campus community from 2020 to 2022), and to implement public-facing digital tools that communicate the potential risk of being exposed and infected by SARS-CoV-2. One of these—the COVID-19 Event Risk Assessment Planning Tool—went "viral" in its own way soon after launch in July 2020, well before vaccines were available. Cumulatively, this tool helped more than 16 million individuals across the country and the world make more than 60 million personalized exposure risk estimates as a means to modify their behavior.

The central premise of our modeling, risk estimation, intervention, and communication efforts is that the number of documented cases has been significantly less than the true number of infections. Collectively, the United States, like other countries, has faced an iceberg-like threat that could be seen only partially by way of documented cases. This gap between the reported and true epidemic burden was partly a consequence of inadequate testing, but it was also a result of something fundamental: the commonplace nature of asymptomatic and mild infections.

In completing this book, I tried to balance the dual aims of communicating as broadly as possible and of revealing the inner workings of the scientific method (and of scientists) when faced with a fast-moving and rapidly evolving threat.

As such, the first part of the book focuses on explaining the governing principles by which asymptomatic transmission can lead to a more severe outbreak at the population scale relative to outbreaks in which transmission is tied to severe symptoms. This was the story of COVID-19.

The second part of the book focuses on practical solutions—specifically, the kinds of data, information landscape, and interventions required to prepare for the danger of pandemics to come. This is the story of what could be.

Building a path toward a better normal will not be straightforward. But effective action requires clear communication of the governing scientific principles that link silent disease spread between individuals to the catastrophic loss of life at population scales.

Whether we heed these lessons remains up to us.

PART I

DECIPHERING THE SILENT SPREAD OF COVID-19

CHAPTER 1

It Was Never Just "the Flu"

Zero Deaths by Summer 2020

On April 13, 2020, Chris Murray, director of the Institute for Health Metrics and Evaluation (IHME), made a bold prediction: COVID-19 deaths in the United States would drop to zero as of June 21, 2020.[1] The claim was backed up by what was apparently a sophisticated computer simulation model of the pandemic. This model was referenced in White House briefings and in situation reports, influencing national policy as well as public understanding of what was to come. At the time, the majority of US states were operating under mandatory stay-at-home orders.[2] Yet the shock of societal change in the face of an unknown threat was already leading to questions. Were such mandates legal? Were they sustainable? Were the public health benefits of locking down people and economies worth the accumulating costs?

The IHME was uniquely positioned to respond to all of these questions. In 2017, the Gates Foundation had set the IHME on course to significantly expand its operations: making a 10-year, $279 million investment in the institute.[3] By 2020, it employed more than 300 staff members, including a range of experts spanning epidemic modeling to economics (as of 2023, the IHME employed more than 500 staff members[4]). This range of expertise was meant to ensure that the IHME would have the capacity to respond to precisely this kind of global pandemic event.

Now was the time to deliver.

Murray explained the rationale for his bold prediction: "We're making this pretty strong assumption that there is no risk of reintroduction post the end of the first wave, however that might come about."[5] In a related part of the interview, when pressed about the mechanism by which deaths would in fact drop to zero, he noted that "the underlying assumption is that something will be put in place—I don't think it's social distancing—that will reduce the risk to essentially zero resurgence."

This claim of a rapid rise and fall in pandemic-induced fatalities was immediately contested by independent experts. In related interviews, Bill Hanage, professor of epidemiology at the Harvard T.H. Chan School of Public Health, put it succinctly: "Unfortunately, there is no way that amount of control could happen by the summer."[6] The IHME model included national and global predictions. The model was equally optimistic about the state of the pandemic worldwide, predicting that the United Kingdom would experience zero COVID-19 deaths after May 31, 2020, multiple weeks earlier than was predicted for the United States. Keith Neal, emeritus professor of epidemiology at the University of Nottingham, offered this pithy take: "Personally, I think the model's pretty useless."[7]

These predictions of zero cases in just a few months amid a devastating spring 2020 wave of infections made national news. Beyond fatalities, the model included estimates of the time course of infections, hospitalizations, and demand in intensive care units (ICUs). The hospitalization data in particular was meant to serve as an early-warning system for state and local public health officials to take the necessary steps to secure ventilators and to avoid overwhelming surges of demand exceeding medical capacity. If the IHME model was flawed, that was a big problem. If the IHME model was useless, that was an even bigger problem.

It turns out that the original IHME model was worse than useless—it was dangerously wrong, providing what appeared to be legitimate cover for an anti-scientific response to a rapidly spreading pandemic.

The reasons are both simple and complicated. The simple reason is that the modelers forgot the cardinal rule of predictions: one is always less sure of the rules underlying complex systems than one thinks. And epidemics are complex systems. The complicated reason is that the IHME model was built on defunct ideas of how epidemics work, not taking into account the ways in which COVID-19 spread and how policymakers and the public reacted to changing pandemic risk.[8]

Figure 1.1 illustrates just how flawed the model was. Released by the IHME as part of its situation reports, the figure reconstructs the IHME model's predictions on April 13, 2020, along with the prior curve of the number of deaths per day in the United States. The gray circles to the left of April 13, 2020 denote the recorded number of COVID-19 fatalities. The dashed line to the right of April 13, 2020, denotes the consensus projection of future fatalities in the IHME model for the subsequent

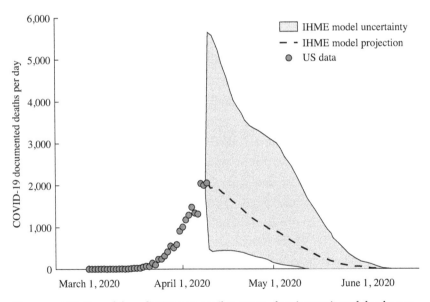

Figure 1.1. IHME model predictions on April 13, 2020, showing projected deaths per day in the United States going to zero by June 13, 2020. The shaded regions denote uncertainty. Hence, the model has high confidence in its prediction of zero deaths. *Source*: IHME COVID-19 health service utilization forecasting team. (2020, March 30). Forecasting COVID-19 impact on hospital bed-days, ICU-days, ventilator days and deaths by US state in the next 4 months. MedRxiv. https://doi.org/10.1101/2020.03.27 .20043752.

three months of the pandemic. In essence, the model assumes that the aggregate effect of lockdowns and physical-distancing interventions put in place in March and April 2020 throughout the United States would be enough to definitively drive down fatalities to zero—in two months. This was not the only bold assertion of the IHME model.

There is a curious feature of the original IHME predictions—which included both a consensus prediction (the dashed line in figure 1.1) and a range of potential scenarios (the shaded region in figure 1.1). The shaded region after April 13, 2020, denotes the ranges in predicted fatalities between mid-April 2020 and the end of June 2020. Notably, the IHME model's prediction has the most uncertainty on its first day. That is, the model seems to be relatively unsure of how many fatalities there might be on April 14, but it is absolutely confident in its prediction of zero fatalities two months into the future. This uncertainty fallacy is a clear indication that the model is flawed. The day-to-day variation suggests that April 14, 2020, was likely going to be a bit worse than April 13, 2020, but not altogether different. This expectation is based on the fact that infections that could have led to fatalities on April 14 were already baked in. Individuals had been infected a few weeks before, and some of these individuals had already progressed to severe illness, had been hospitalized, or perhaps had already been intubated. Moreover, precisely because COVID-19 was an emerging infectious disease spreading within an immunologically naive population, there was little to no scientific rationale for thinking that the disease could disappear nearly as fast as it arose. As a result, there should be some level of uncertainty at the beginning of a model prediction and even more uncertainty two or three months hence.

To paraphrase Yogi Berra: it's tough to make predictions, especially about the future.

Despite the impression that the IHME had a sophisticated model driving its forecasts, these original predictions were not based on a state-of-the-art mechanistic model of infection. A mechanistic model tries to understand the underlying reasons for a disease's spread—and then extrapolates into the future. A mechanistic model would take into account how many people were susceptible to infection, how many were infected, and how many had recovered. The model would then try—however difficult it may be—to build a forecast from the estimated disease state of the population. Indeed, a principled model would have tried to account for the interactions between susceptible and infectious individuals leading to new infections; it would have tried to account for the recovery of infectious individuals as well as for changes in behavior, the impact of policy changes, and perhaps even the thorny problems of community structure, undertesting, and underreporting. The fact that many cases were never identified is one critical reason why early epidemic models were so hard to calibrate. For example, if one were to try and gauge an epidemic model's performance against case counts, then immediately something would appear to have gone wrong either with the model or with the data itself. Let's explore why.

By mid-April 2020, the United States was experiencing more than 2,000 COVID-19 fatalities per day.[9] Yet early estimates from Wuhan, China, suggested that the infection fatality rate (the fraction of infected individuals who die) was approximately 1 in 100 or perhaps 1 in 200.[10] These fatalities typically occurred a few weeks post-infection because of the progression of the disease and efforts to intubate and save those most severely infected. In aggregate, there is typically a two- to three-week difference between exposure, onset of symptoms, hospitalization, and death for COVID-19. As a result, if the United States had 2,000 new COVID-19 fatalities per day in mid-April, then there should have been 200,000 new infections per day in late March or early April 2020 (a factor 100-times greater). The reported case count was far less. Instead, there had only been 15,000 to 25,000 cases reported per day in the United States by late March and early April 2020.[11] Reconciling observed levels of hospitalization and fatalities with documented case reports required that some other mechanism may be in play.

For scientists, it is essential to explore potential alternative hypotheses when confronted with data that seems inconsistent. For example, here are two ways to think about the gap between expected cases and observed cases of COVID-19.

Hypothesis 1—SARS-CoV-2 is far worse than expected at the individual level

This hypothesis assumes that finding 15,000 to 25,000 cases rather than 200,000 cases means that SARS-CoV-2 was far more likely to cause severe illness or death in those infected than prior studies out of Wuhan had suggested. If this were true, then perhaps the chance of dying from infection (i.e., the infection fatality rate) was closer to 10% than 1% or 0.5%. Yet such a hypothesis implies that the SARS-CoV-2 strains circulating in the United States, the US population, or some combination of both were fundamentally different from those in Wuhan—and more likely to lead to severe outcomes. This hypothesis seemed far-fetched, especially in light of the significant number of asymptomatic infections. As a result, the reaction of most epidemic modeling groups was to turn to a different hypothesis.

Hypothesis 2—The vast majority of COVID-19 cases were not documented

This hypothesis assumes that the SARS-CoV-2 strains spreading in the United States were largely equivalent in terms of their transmissibility to those that emerged in Wuhan. Moreover, this hypothesis assumes that the age-specific risk of death was similar regardless of geographic locale. (Variants and evolution are issues of importance later in this book.) Hence, the gap in expected cases versus reported cases points to a failure to find cases rather than to a change in the virus or the population. At the early stages of the pandemic, the testing system was so inadequate and hampered by the prevalence of asymptomatic infections that the United States was likely discovering only 1 in 10 cases.[12] This failure to find cases—driven by inadequate testing and asymptomatic infections—presented challenges to epidemic simulation models. Moreover, if COVID-19 frequently led to asymptomatic outcomes (i.e., mild infections, infections without symptoms specifically associated with COVID-19, or the absence of symptoms altogether), then it would be very hard to identify who should be tested, especially given limited testing capacity.

There are many ways to deal with such missing data. One way would be to infer the missing cases by assuming an infection fatality rate and moving backward in time. By taking current hospitalization and/or fatality rates, models could then look backward in time and compare the documented number of cases with the expected number of cases. The gap between them represents the ascertainment bias. Hence, if one expected to find 10,000 cases/day a few weeks ago and there were only 2,000 reported cases/day, then one can infer that the ascertainment bias is five: that is, only one in five cases was identified and reported to public health authorities. A high ascertainment bias means that the vast majority of infections are not found. By including underreporting, it is possible to calibrate epidemic models so that they can reconcile infections, hospitalizations, and deaths. And when a model is calibrated correctly, the actual number of infections in the community can be a clue for understanding the speed of population-level transmission into the future. But this is not what the IHME model did. Instead, it inadvertently repeated a mistake from more than a century ago.

The Misuse of Farr's "Law" of Epidemics

The IHME model was built on hope. Hope is good. In many stages of the pandemic, hope has been on our side. Look at the speed at which mRNA vaccines were developed, tested, scaled up, and delivered to (some) of the world. But in public health crises, one should hope for the best and prepare for the worst.[13] Instead, early versions of the IHME model hoped for the best and then doubled-down on hope. Despite the investment, despite the large staff, despite visualizations that connected past data to future projections, the underlying mathematical model that drove the IHME simulation was a curve fit—and not in a good sense.

The IHME built its early forecasts predicting the rapid decline of COVID-19 cases on a curve with a long history. The curve is a special kind of mathematical function called "erf" (known colloquially among statisticians as the error function).[14] The error function has many uses and an attractive property: it can fit shapes that go up rapidly and then just as rapidly come to a halt. In other words, what the IHME model did was to aggregate recent deaths, add them up to get a cumulative curve, and then assume that the curve would soon flatten as new deaths vanished. Such curve fitting can look good in the moment. But if one projects such curve fits into the future, they tend to fail, miserably. The failure is even worse insofar as this kind of mistake has been made many times before—with predictably similar outcomes.

The fact that the IHME model assumed that the curve would flatten soon is a consequence of a deeper assumption akin to taking a bell-shaped curve for epidemics. The IHME model assumed that epidemics inevitably rise and fall symmetrically. For example, if it takes four weeks from the first case for an epidemic to peak, then it should take four weeks for the disease to vanish. Moreover, if the epidemic case curve is beginning to show signs of saturating, then the erf model interprets this saturation as a harbinger of a downturn, eventually leading to the predictable end of the epidemic.

The idea that diseases spread in a pattern of symmetric rises and falls has its origins in a defunct epidemiological "law" called Farr's law. William Farr was a nineteenth-century physician who was instrumental in the development of medical statistics, often in the context of responding to smallpox outbreaks. In 1839, he observed that smallpox "destroyed more than 30,819 persons" in England.[15] Understanding and controlling the spread of smallpox was of utmost necessity. Farr looked carefully at death records throughout the country and observed that when focusing on a particular region, the outbreak size seemed to change in a regular fashion. He posed the following quandary in his 1839 report: "Why do the five deaths become 10, 15, 20, 31, 58, 88 weekly, and then progressively fall through the same measured steps." Was there in fact a principle that determines how disease burden goes up and down?

Farr's answer was to propose that there were hidden features of the spread of disease within individuals and within a population that drove a symmetric outbreak—one that went up and down at essentially the same speed. This insight is valuable—especially as a starting point.

Some diseases do exhibit such symmetry, or nearly so. Science is not static, however. The insights of 150 years ago represent a partial understanding of how diseases work; remarkably, they precede the development of the central postulates of what causes disease (i.e., germs or pathogens[16]) and the first visualization of viruses under a microscope (which took place in the late 1930s[17]).

Nonetheless, Farr's observations were revived in 1990 in a paper published in the *Journal of the American Medical Association* as part of an effort to try and predict the potential for the emerging AIDS epidemic to spread both nationally and globally.[18] The authors of the study used the initial rise of AIDS cases as a means to predict future incidence, year by year. Because the case data exhibited a slight decrease in its rate of increase between 1985 and 1987, they interpreted this change as an indication that the symmetric Farr's law would soon take over and that cases would fall just as fast as they had risen. Figure 1.2 is a reproduction of their predictions.

The authors used Farr's law, fit the case data, and made the bold prediction in 1990 that "the projected size of the [AIDS] epidemic falls in the range of 200,000 cases and effectively ends by the mid 1990s."[19] Nothing could be further from the truth. In 1995 alone, there were more than 500,000 confirmed AIDS diagnoses in the United States, with no signs of abating.[20] There have been more than 40 million deaths globally from AIDS. And HIV (human immunodeficiency virus, which leads to AIDS) remains a global threat even now—despite the benefits of antiviral drugs that can help stabilize infections, provided those drugs are accessible to those who need them.[21] Yet, for all the apparent technical sophistication, the IHME model used a variant of this same defunct epidemiological "law."

Some epidemic outbreaks do exhibit nearly symmetric up-and-down patterns. But there is no a priori reason why they must. In fact, there is far more evidence that they do not, especially in the case of an emerging infectious disease spreading in an immunologically naive population. The use of a curve-fitting function also explains why the IHME model seemed to gain (false) confidence about the future. If one has a series of points in a cumulative death trajectory and tries to fit a curve

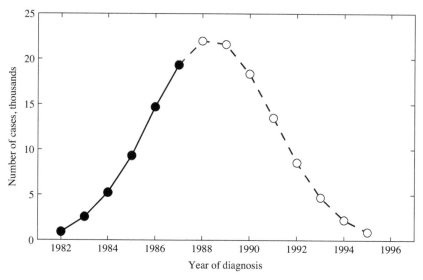

Figure 1.2. A prediction of the annual incidence of AIDS in the United States using data between 1982 and 1987 (solid circles) and projecting forward through 1995 using Farr's law (open circles). The actual number of newly confirmed US-based AIDS cases in 1995 exceeded 75,000, nearly four times higher than the number of cases in 1987. *Source*: Redrawn with data from figure 2 of Bregman, D.J., and Langmuir, A.D. (1990). Farr's law applied to AIDS projections. *JAMA* 263: 1522–1525. https://doi.org/10.1001/jama.1990.03440110088033.

to it, then inevitably there will be some uncertainty at the start. Moreover, the very nature of the erf curve fit forces new cases to drop to zero while forcing the cumulative cases to plateau. This kind of model fit excludes the possibility of a rebound and does not permit the possibility of different shapes (like sustained nonzero levels of deaths per day during a long plateau period). Over time, the IHME model did change its near-term predictions, upwardly revising death estimates as the pandemic did not end as predicted. When its predictions changed, certain public-facing statistical experts seemed to think that the model's approach was sound. On April 17, 2020, Nate Silver tweeted out the following observation: "Model outputs *should* change in response to new data and when you're dealing with nonlinear systems, small changes can have a reasonably large effect."[22]

This tweet—even at the time—reflected a misunderstanding of what the IHME was doing. It was not modeling a nonlinear "system" (complex or otherwise); it was fitting curves to a series of points. And when the points updated (because new data came in that deviated from prior predictions), then the curves were readjusted, always pointing back toward zero a few months in the future. This did not make the model outputs sensible; it simply reinforced the problematic nature of the IHME's approach. The IHME model kept predicting a symmetric up-and-down shape, even as the data kept defying the very assumptions built into the model. Unfortunately, the IHME model was certainly not the only example of premature declarations of "mission accomplished."

In early May 2020, news reports revealed that President Donald Trump's administration was using an epidemic model developed by White House economic advisor Kevin Hassett as part of its pandemic assessment and response. This model predicted that COVID 19 cases would drop to zero in as few as 10 days.[23] What expertise in epidemic analysis did Hassett have? Little to none. Like the IHME model, this prediction was not based on trying to ascertain the way that SARS-CoV-2 was spreading between individuals or how different reactions to lockdowns might change the future course of the epidemic. Instead, Hassett's epidemic model consisted of taking recent case data and fitting the data to a "cubic" function using the built-in function in an Excel spreadsheet.[24]

Cubic functions are convenient ways to visualize rapid ups and downs in a data series. They are a step up in complexity from a quadratic function, which itself is a step up in complexity from a line. A quadratic function makes a shape like a bowl and can be oriented in two directions, either right side up so that you could place fruit in it or upside down so that fruit would roll off it onto the floor. A cubic function connects two oppositely oriented fruit bowls together. This means that it can be a nice way to try and fit data that has a roller-coaster-like property—going up and down and then up again or, alternatively, going down and up and then down again. If one does not span the entire scope of predictions, then a cubic can look like a quadratic (or a line). But one thing a cubic cannot do is keep oscillating. And so, over the long term, it doesn't even make sense to think about the cubic function as an epidemic model. A cubic model, like Farr's law, is a curve fit. Because of the double-fruit-bowl effect, when applied to epidemic data, cubic-function fits must ultimately predict either infinitely many or zero cases. Hassett chose the version of the model that corresponded to a rapid convergence to zero cases. This prediction was nonsensical, even more so in light of what occurred later.

Both IHME's erf model and Hassett's cubic model saw the end as inevitable. It could be that some intervention was possible that could stop the epidemic in its tracks—yet at the time, vaccines were not on the near-term horizon. Alternatively, perhaps so many individuals were being infected with mild or asymptomatic cases that some process would drive cases to zero and help them stay there. This type of wishful thinking could not have been more misguided.

These failures hold a kernel of understanding. Both the erf and cubic model reflect confusion with how to grapple with the gap between the large number of fatalities and the relatively small number of cases. Something was missing in the data. Precisely because it was so hard to measure the extent of infections, perhaps this early wave came with an even larger, hidden wave of asymptomatic and undocumented cases. If so, perhaps the pandemic would be over soon. Such hope seemed attractive, certainly more so than the alternative. One of the reasons why curve-fit models could gain credibility is that there was in fact significant asymptomatic spread—just not nearly as much as either model assumed. That idea and story spread to our collective detriment, and in far too many instances, the story drove some to avoid taking precautions (or later, to avoid vaccines) and so die for (or because of) a misinformed belief. At the core of this misinformed belief was confusion over just how frequently individuals died after having contracted SARS-CoV-2 and how such fatality rates should influence pandemic response.

Misestimation of Fatality Rates in the First Wave

On February 19, 2020, two soccer teams competed in the UEFA Champions League match held on a winter's evening at the San Siro stadium, a few miles outside Milan's city center. The Round of 16 game between Atalanta (from northeast Italy, close to Milan) and Valencia (from the southeast coast of Spain) was a critical step in the months-long process to be crowned the best soccer team in Europe. It also accelerated the spread and dispersal of COVID-19 throughout the region.[25] The result, a 4–1 win for Atalanta, was soon overshadowed. The first documented case of COVID-19 in the region was identified on February 20. The region of ~10 million individuals had full-scale lockdowns by early March, leaving residents unable to leave towns and villages (though many did get out, fleeing the lockdowns and, in many instances, taking the virus with them), even as the care of the sick was undermined by Lombardy's withered hospital system, a result of prior privatization marked by corruption.[26]

By April 15, 2020, less than two months after the Champions League match, the Lombardy region had documented more than 11,000 fatalities from COVID-19, approximately one-half that of the entire country, despite having only one-sixth of the population. Taken at face value, the case severity and fatality rate in Lombardy seemed improbably high.[27] In late February and early March 2020, approximately 50% of positive cases were hospitalized and approximately 20% required treatment in an ICU. Moreover, the 11,000 fatalities were attributed to approximately 60,000 documented cases—implying a case fatality rate approaching 20%. These levels were significantly higher than those estimated in Wuhan and again suggested that either COVID-19 had an enormously high risk of causing fatalities (approaching that of smallpox) or the vast majority of cases had never been identified.

This latter idea—that asymptomatic spread was rampant—helped explain the gap between cases and deaths, but it also suggested another possibility. What happened if case ascertainment was really, really poor? What if the ratio between actual infections and reported cases at the start of the pandemic was not just 10 but 20, 50, or even 100. That is, if the ascertainment bias was on the order of 100, then the Lombardy region's infection fatality rate must be calculated as the ratio of fatalities to actual, rather than documented, infections. Hence, rather than dividing 11,377 by 62,153 (the number of documented cases as of April 15, 2020), one should divide 11,377 by 6,215,300 (the number of infections by that same date, assuming only 1 in 100 infections were ascertained). If that were the case, then there would be two enormously relevant consequences:

1. COVID-19 was no worse than the flu, with an infection fatality rate close to 0.1% (or perhaps even lower).
2. More than 50% of the population had already been infected; that is, the pandemic was nearly over, as the virus would soon run out of new individuals to infect.

Both of these ideas turned out to be wrong—and there was already enough evidence to reach that conclusion at the time such ideas were proposed. But this line of thought was precisely the one adopted by an influential group of Stanford University–based medical doctors, scientists, and economists. Such thinking addressed a legitimate uncertainty driven by asymptomatic infections. If we did not have the testing capacity to identify the vast sea of infections amid the relatively few symptomatic cases, then debating the extent of missing infections was important. Yet the debate was not between whether we were missing 9 of 10 or 4 of 5 infections—instead, proponents of the idea that COVID-19 was no worse than the flu began to suggest that public health authorities were missing 99 out of 100 infections or even 299 out of 300 infections.

It is instructive to revisit the perspective of one of the foremost advocates for a proposal that COVID-19 was no worse than the flu. On March 17, 2020, Dr. John Ioannidis, a well-known physician-scientist at Stanford University, wrote an opinion piece for the news website STAT.[28] Most Americans do not rank STAT up there with *USA Today*, the *Washington Post*, or the *New York Times*. Many have never even heard of STAT—indeed, many scientists have not heard of it either. But, for those working in health and medicine, STAT is a widely recognized and reputable outlet, one based in the *Boston Globe*'s offices.[29] In fact, STAT staff and contributing reporters had already put out thoughtful coverage of the COVID-19 pandemic.

Ioannidis's opinion piece was titled "A Fiasco in the Making? As the Coronavirus Pandemic Takes Hold, We Are Making Decisions without Reliable Data." The author's first premise was that the data was unreliable. This was true, to some extent. In Ioannidis's terms:

> The data collected so far on how many people are infected and how the epidemic is evolving are utterly unreliable. Given the limited testing to date, some deaths and probably the vast majority of infections due to SARS-CoV-2 are being missed. We don't know if we are failing to capture infections by a factor of three or 300. Three months after the outbreak emerged, most countries, including the U.S., lack the ability to test a large number of people and no countries have reliable data on the prevalence of the virus in a representative random sample of the general population.[30]

By this stage, there had been only a few detailed studies of infection fatality rates to comprehensively examine the severity of COVID-19. One example was the outbreak on the *Diamond Princess* cruise ship.[31] The cruise ship had set sail from the port of Yokohama in Japan on January 20, 2020. By February 1, it was clear there was a problem: multiple individuals had confirmed symptoms, and one of the earliest individuals to get sick tested positive for SARS-CoV-2. The shipboard outbreak eventually led to more than 600 infections among the ~3,700 passengers and crew within three weeks of the first documented case, for an infection rate of nearly 20%. The ship was quarantined off the coast for weeks before passengers (and later the crew) were finally allowed to disembark. Of those infected, seven had died by March 17, and although exact figures and direct links of infection became more difficult to determine after individuals left the ship, the total number of fatalities attributable to COVID-19 implied a case fatality rate of around 2.6% and an infection fatality rate of approximately 1.3%.[32] Here, the case fatality rate (the fraction of documented cases who died) and the infection fatality rate (the fraction of infected individuals who died) were thought to be close, because systematic testing of those aboard left less room for missed infections. These fatality rate estimates were made public on March 9, 2020.[33] But Ioannidis was not deterred.

Perhaps the high fatality rates on the *Diamond Princess* had been influenced by the age demographics of typical cruise-going passengers compared with the population overall. The age distribution of those aboard winter cruises in Japan does not reflect the entire society—like in the United States, cruise takers tend to be older than the average age of the populace. The data from Wuhan had already demonstrated that the risk of fatality increased with age (an issue to be examined in detail in the next section). Hence, Ioannidis argued that "projecting the Diamond Princess mortality rate onto the age structure of the U.S. population, the death rate among people infected with COVID-19 would be 0.125%."[34] The value of 0.125% is equivalent to 1 death per 800 infections. If true in Lombardy, this would imply that the 11,000 documented fatalities by mid-April correspond to nearly 11,000 × 800, or ~9 million, infections in a population of approximately 10 million. In other words, the outbreak should have come to a rapid halt as the virus ran out of anyone else to infect.

Ioannidis extrapolated the range of potential outcomes for the infection fatality rate to lie within 0.05% to 1%. This range is equivalent to saying that anywhere from a minimum of 1 in 2,000 infections leads to a fatality (0.05%) to a maximum of 1 in 100 infections (1%). A few days after Ioannidis published his article, Dr. Scott Atlas—another scholar affiliated with the Hoover Institution at Stanford University and a White House COVID-19 advisor—reached out to Seema Verma, the administrator of the Centers for Medicare and Medicaid Services, highlighting the prediction that only 10,000 individuals would die in a COVID-19 pandemic. Atlas's central point was that if one were to use estimates from the middle of Ioannidis's range, then cumulative COVID-19 deaths would go "unnoticed" in the total of flu-like deaths every season.[35]

As of March 2022, the United States crossed the threshold of 1 million fatalities from COVID-19 in a population of approximately 330 million.[36] Evolution of strains notwithstanding, it is essentially impossible for the effective population-level infection fatality rate in immunologically naive individuals to be less than 1/330, or 0.3%. This level is nearly 10 times greater than the estimate that Ioannidis used for his initial assessment. There are not enough individuals in the entire United States to account for some of the lower ranges of infection fatality rates. But, one might argue, we did not know that for a year (or more) after Ioannidis's essay in Stat.

In fact, evidence from Wuhan and Lombardy (and New York City) would make something clear by March and April 2020: COVID-19 was not the flu.

Seasonal flu does not lead to the sound of ambulance sirens heard day and night in cities. Seasonal flu does not lead to an overflow in hospital ICUs or the accumulation of the dead to the point that mobile morgues are required to accommodate the bodies.[37,38] Seasonal flu does not cause more than 10,000 deaths in Lombardy (with a population the size of the state of Georgia) in less than two months[39] and does not cause more than 20,000 deaths in New York City in the single month of April 2020.[40] The vast majority of public health experts with an understanding of the potential speed and severity of SARS-CoV-2's spread had made their warnings clear: this was not the flu. Instead, catastrophic spread was altogether possible. Yet, rather than take the middle range of his own estimates, Ioannidis made extreme assumptions, including the possibility that only 1 in 2,000 COVID-19 infections would lead to a fatality. He warned his readers accordingly: "A population-wide case fatality rate of 0.05% is lower than seasonal influenza. If that is the true rate, locking down the world with potentially tremendous social and financial consequences may be totally irrational. It's like an elephant being attacked by a house cat. Frustrated and trying to avoid the cat, the elephant accidentally jumps off a cliff and dies."[41]

Of course, COVID-19 was no house cat.

In his defense, Ioannidis did propose one way to cut through some of the confusion—by pointing to the critical need to use a different kind of test to estimate the cumulative number of infections. The need for another approach is paramount when symptoms are not a reliable barometer for an infection. Testing for virus can be used for many reasons: as a means to confirm a diagnosis, to try and short-circuit the spread of illness when individuals have had close contact with a confirmed positive case, and perhaps even systematically to identify and isolate individuals to reduce the spread of disease. Each of these has a value, and testing is a key focus in the latter half of this book on mechanisms to sustain a victory against COVID and pandemics to come. But the one thing viral testing cannot necessarily do is provide a measure of whether someone *previously* had an infection.

Testing for Signs of Viral Presence and Past

Given the inadequacy of viral testing and the potential for asymptomatic spread in early 2020, it was essential to try and estimate how many people had already been infected in the United States with SARS-CoV-2. But how does one go backward in time and figure out who had been infected if they were never tested for an infection in the first place? To answer this question requires leveraging the time course of a SARS-CoV-2 infection within an individual. After exposure and infection, individuals infected with SARS-CoV-2 will experience no symptoms, at least at first. This period is known as the "exposed" or "incubation" phase. For SARS-CoV-2, that exposed period can be as few as two to three days but can also extend to six days (or beyond).[42] During this incubation period, the SARS-CoV-2 viruses are replicating within cells—starting with nasal, tracheal, and lung epithelial cells, then moving potentially to other cells in different organs, whether in the gastrointestinal tract, cardiovascular system, testes, kidney, or even thyroid cells.[43] (Note: the varied cells and organs infected by SARS-CoV-2 is one indication of the ways in which COVID-19 is not just a respiratory illness.) When the viral load in the body remains relatively low, then standard molecular viral tests may not be able to detect a signal.

Viral tests—also known as reverse transcription polymerase chain reaction (RT-PCR) tests—work by taking a sample and then adding enzymes that turn viral RNA inside the sample into a strand of DNA (i.e., a single strand of the famous double helix structure).[44] Then, many complementary strands of a target piece of DNA are added to the sample so that if SARS-CoV-2 is present, the original single helix will become a double helix—at least in a specific part. Then, the test cycles through high and low temperatures to separate out the double helix into single helices, and then by flooding the sample with the target piece of DNA, the single helices can become double helices again. Eventually, there are so many of these double helices that a small presence of SARS-CoV-2 RNA in a saliva or nose swab sample can become detectable. Yet, there are limits. If there is no (or too little) SARS-CoV-2 RNA in the sample, then the target pieces in the test will have nothing to bind to, and there will be no amplification and no signal. For this reason, viral tests of infected individuals can be negative if tests are taken too early after exposure.

As viral load increases, then the chances of a positive test from a small sample taken from saliva or the nasal passageway increases rapidly, nearly to 100%. This positive PCR signal can persist for many days, if not up to a week (or two) after the incubation phase. There are even rarer cases of individuals who test PCR positive for weeks after an infection. Yet this does not necessarily mean that an individual remains infectious. PCR tests for the presence of viral RNA. But viral RNA alone is not confirmatory evidence of the existence of *infectious* viral particles. A gold-standard test would be to take a sample and try to grow the viruses in a cell culture. This is extremely laborious and infeasible to scale up as a public health intervention. Instead, it is possible to search for signatures of the virus particle itself. The idea is that an individual who is infectious will be actively shedding virus particles—containing both viral RNA as well as proteins that form the shell and "body" of the virus (see the glossary for more information on the components of SARS-CoV-2 virus particles). Viral proteins can be recognized by the immune system, but they can also be recognized rapidly through low-cost antigen tests (figure 1.3).

The principle of such antigen tests is to use small filter strips preloaded with antibodies to bind and signal the presence of SARS-CoV-2 virus particles. Antibodies are proteins expressed by specialized parts of the immune system in response to an infection—like that of SARS-CoV-2. These antibodies are quite specific, recognizing only specific kinds of foreign pathogens. Hence, by preloading antibodies specific

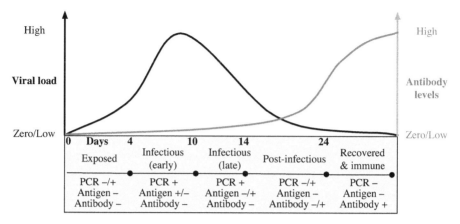

Figure 1.3. Schematic of the relationship between viral load (left y-axis), antibody levels (right y-axis), disease status (below x-axis), and test status (below disease status). There are multiple kinds of antibodies; here, the schematic depicts the trajectory of more durable IgG antibodies.

to the spike protein found on the surface of the SARS-CoV-2 virus particle, it is possible to take a small saliva or nasal-swab sample and add it on the surface of these preloaded strips as a means to detect the presence of viral "antigens" (i.e., parts of the spike proteins). Antigens can be thought of as keys that open the door to cells. Antibodies are mobile locks that circulate outside the cells. These antibodies can bind viral antigens, preventing the entry of virus particles into cells. The same principle can be used in an antigen test. In this case, antibodies preloaded on the strip will bind to the viral antigens. Enough of these binding events cause these key-lock aggregates to form clusters; antibody binding to targets leads to the telltale bright red line found on pregnancy tests and on SARS-CoV-2 rapid tests. These positive antigen tests indicate that the individual is shedding virus—presumably infectious virus. Antigen tests will also be discussed in later chapters focusing on the use of testing as a form of mitigation.[45]

John Ioannidis speculated that the vast majority of individuals infected with SARS-CoV-2 were never identified. The fraction of asymptomatic infection was thought to be high, and combined with the paucity of testing, it was at least plausible to think that back in the period between January and April 2020, the vast majority of infections would remain undetected. If that were so, then there should be a way to find hidden infections—not by using PCR or even antigen tests but instead by using a test to look for the residue of an infection: antibodies.

A typical antibody test is more complicated to perform than standard PCR or antigen tests that probe for the presence of viral RNA or viral particles, respectively. Here, the test must search for evidence that an individual has circulating antibodies specific to a target. The presence of antibodies indicates that the individual is producing many "locks," and these can be identified using a lab test that mixes these locks with an appropriate key. In practice, a blood draw is performed, and then the blood sampled is mixed with viral antigens (though some researchers have managed to develop similar tests using saliva).[46] These viral antigens are typically spike proteins from the SARS-CoV-2 virus. A positive test signal means that the serum sample had antibodies, which in turn means that the individual who donated the sample almost certainly had a prior infection. If enough people's blood sera could be collected and tested in an unbiased fashion, then it might be possible to estimate the true number of prior infections, compare it to the known number of infections documented through viral tests, and estimate the ascertainment bias.

This procedure takes work. But the outcome has the potential to tell us how many people had been infected and, in turn, estimate the infection fatality rate—that is, the ratio of the number of documented fatalities to the total number of infections (including asymptomatic infections).

The only problem was that no such systematic studies of antibody levels in the population had been conducted. At least not yet, and that was about to change.

The Santa Clara Serological Survey

From April 3 to April 4, 2020, a team of Bay Area scientists, led by Dr. Eran Bendavid and Dr. Jay Bhattacharya of Stanford Medical School (and including Ioannidis) sampled residents of Santa Clara County, recruiting individuals through Facebook ads and word-of-mouth. Individuals had to drive to one of three test collection sites, sign a consent form that stated they understood the study purpose, and then donate blood sera to be analyzed using a standard serological assay kit designed to test for antibodies to SARS-CoV-2. The results—as described—appeared startling.[47]

The team tried to account for variability in test performance as well as for what they considered to be potential biases in the representative sample of more than 3,000 participants. In doing so, they estimated that between 2.5% to 4.2% of residents had a prior infection. In retrospect, this might seem low, considering the cumulative frequency of SARS-CoV-2 infections during the pandemic. At the time, however, these estimated levels were 50 to 85 times higher than concurrent estimates for Santa Clara County. This level of prior infection also implied that raw case fatality rates should be downgraded by a factor of between 50 to 85 times—just as Ioannidis had speculated (in the absence of direct evidence) a month before. If correct and applied both in the United States and globally, the findings heralded that COVID-19 was, to borrow Ioannidis term, just a house cat; moreover, the end of the pandemic was near.

To understand the implications of a finding that only 1 in 50 or 1 in 85 cases was documented, let us again revisit the Lombardy region of Italy. As previously detailed, Milan and the adjoining region were particularly hard hit in the earliest phase of the COVID-19 pandemic. By April 15, more than 11,000 individuals had died of COVID-19 in Lombardy, despite the fact that the health authorities had only documented ~63,000 cases—implying that nearly 20% of every documented case led to a fatality. But, what if Ioannidis, Bendavid, Bhattacharya, and colleagues were correct? If one assumes that authorities in Lombardy were only able to documented 1 in 50 or 1 in 85 cases, then those 63,000 documented cases were actually associated with between 3 million to 5 million infections out of a population of approximately 10 million. If true, the COVID-19 infection fatality rate would be something closer to 0.2%—approaching that of seasonal flu.

On April 17, 2020, these results were posted to academic preprint servers meant to accelerate dissemination of scientific findings.[48] The findings immediately began to influence state and national-level policy.[49,50] If these results held, then it implied that the asymptomatic infection route was not only as frequent as the symptomatic infection route—it was far, far larger. And, if most infections were asymptomatic, then many more people might become infected, but the vast majority of them would not get sick or die. Taking the logic a step further, if the asymptomatic infection fraction was sufficiently high, then the population as a whole might be closer to reaching what is termed a "herd immunity" level of prior infections (an issue we will return to in later chapters). With so many people already infected, it is harder for the disease to spread. The aggregate result would be a rapid rise in fatalities (largely among the vulnerable and elderly) followed by a rapid crash. Hence, if all of this were true, then one should expect the end of the pandemic was near, and the total level of fatalities for COVID-19 was going to turn out to be no different from that arising from seasonal flu.

But none of this was true.

Ioannidis is a prolific author. Writing fast does not necessarily mean that what is written stands the test of time. Ioannidis had cautioned precisely against the frantic push to publish. One of his most famous contributions is a paper that concluded that most published research findings are false.[51] The article was published in a prestigious medical sciences journal (known familiarly as *PLOS Medicine*) and has been cited more than 10,000 times. In other words, more than 10,000 other scientific articles relied, in part, on Ioannidis's work on the false nature of research as the basis for their own studies. In baseball terms, that's a Ruthian level of impact. Ioannidis central claim is that the incentive to publish positive results inevitably leads scientists to look for statistically significant evidence in their experiments. Eventually, scientists find a level of evidence that will withstand the critique of peer reviewers and submit their results to academic journals, which eventually accept and publish the findings. But this frantic push to publish ultimately undermines the power of the findings—given that if one asks enough questions of the data, one will eventually find a "statistically significant" pattern.

The scientific preprint documenting the findings of the Santa Clara serological study immediately received intense pushback and critique.[52] The critiques focused predominantly on two issues: (i) the effectiveness of the test and (ii) the unbiased nature of the sample. Designing unbiased samples of a population is nontrivial, and the importance of reaching the entire public when implementing public health interventions will be addressed in part 2 of this book. But, for now, it is sufficient to revisit the Santa Clara serological study through the lens of medical test statistics.

Understanding what went wrong with the serological study requires understanding something about the challenges of estimating the frequency of a relatively rare condition in a population using an imperfect test. And the tests in the Santa Clara study were not perfect—no test is. Indeed, even high-quality tests sometimes give positive results when the individual's condition is negative, and vice versa. In this case, the study team decided to use a "lateral flow immunological assay" technology. But the details of the assay and the (poor) quality of early serological tests are perhaps secondary to a fundamental statistical fallacy. The assay used was reported to have had an approximate 99% specificity and perhaps 80% sensitivity. That seems very good, but it turns out that neglecting the real possibility of false positives undermines the confidence in the serological findings.

How good is a medical test with 99% specificity and 80% sensitivity? The answer depends on context.

The term *specificity* denotes the chance that an individual who is negative for the condition will return a negative test result. Hence, if someone did not previously have COVID-19, then an antibody test with 99% specificity would return a negative test result 99/100 times. But, the same test would return a positive test result 1/100 times. This one test result in a pool of 100 individuals who never had the disease, then, is a false positive. Likewise, the term *sensitivity* denotes the chance that an individual who is positive for the condition will return a positive test result. Hence, if someone did have COVID, then a test with

80% sensitivity would return a positive result 80/100 times. But, the same test would return a negative test result 20/100 times. Those 20 results are false negatives.

That seems relatively good, but not if the actual frequency of the condition (in this case, having previously had COVID) was also rare. It is instructive to think about a population in which 2 people out of 100 have, in fact, had COVID. All 100 people are then tested. Given the 80% sensitive test, it is likely that both individuals who had COVID return positive test results. But there are still 98 others to test (and the test designers do not know their prior disease status). Because of the 99% specificity, we expect approximately 1 false positive out of this cohort. Hence, when sampling a population of 100, we end up with 3 positives, including 1 false positive. Even worse, if only one person had previously had COVID, it is likely that the sample would return 2 positive test results; of these, only 1 would be a true positive—so a 50% chance of a false positive!

We can extend this idea to a population of 3,000 and consider a case in which approximately 20 people were found to have previously had COVID. The group of 3,000 represents 30 blocks of 100 individuals. Yet, in each block, it is possible that one individual would have a false positive test because of the specificity of the use of the lateral flow technology. Adding those up could lead to approximately 30 false positive cases. Given the sensitivity, perhaps only 15 to 20 true-positive cases would be found, for a total of 50 positive cases. Depending on the sample size, it is plausible to think that the majority of "positive" test results even in a population with little to no actual history of prior COVID-19 infection. This is precisely the reaction of other experts. For example, as Mark Kilpatrick noted, "With that false positive rate, a large number of the positive cases reported in the study—50 out of 3300 tests—could be false positives."[53]

It is plausible that the Santa Clara study overestimated the infection prevalence by a factor of 10, because the researchers did not sufficiently account for false positives. In fact, one cannot rule out the possibility that no one in the entire sample previously had COVID-19. Even if that is an extreme assumption, it is more likely that the Santa

Clara County findings could be interpreted to mean that there were between 5 and 8.5 more infections than documented cases, rather than between 50 and 85. Yet that is precisely what the public health community had been saying at the outset. It meant that the population of Santa Clara, and California, and the United States (and Italy and China, and everywhere else) remained almost entirely immunologically naive, that infection fatality rates were close to 1%, and that if the disease were to spread to 50% or more of the population, then there would be large-scale illness, hospitalizations, and fatalities. That scenario is what unfolded.

Taking the right steps in spring 2020 required being realistic about the COVID-19 threat. While many scientists and public health experts were aware of the threat, the Santa Clara study presented a counterargument that helped fuel confusion and misinformation. Ultimately, any evaluation of these competing narratives requires looking retrospectively at a key barometer of harm: the contrasting death rates of COVID-19 and the flu.

Deaths Rates from COVID-19 and the Flu

COVID-19 spreading in an immunologically naive population is different from seasonal flu—fundamentally different. Seasonal influenza does not lead to overwhelmed hospitals, mobile morgues, and the sustained and synchronized spread of illness and large-scale fatalities at a pace that was apparent in Wuhan, the Lombardy region in Italy, and in the urban centers of the Northeast United States in early 2020. Yet, with hindsight, it is possible to elaborate on the ways in which the cumulative severity of COVID-19 does or does not compare to that of the flu.[54]

Let us start by contrasting documented death rates. Table 1.1 summarizes reports from the Centers for Disease Control and Prevention (CDC) on the number of COVID deaths, influenza deaths, and total deaths for different age groups over an approximately two-year period, beginning in January 2020 and concluding in March 2022.

In this period, there were nearly 1 million documented fatalities from COVID-19 and approximately 10,000 documented fatalities

Table 1.1. Aggregate COVID-19 vs. influenza deaths, with relative death risk ratio and total deaths, by age group

Age Group	COVID Deaths	Influenza Deaths	COVID:Influenza Death Risk Ratio	Total Deaths (all causes)
<1 year	224	27	8.3	40,604
1–4 years	101	67	1.5	7,562
5–14 years	268	81	3.3	12,071
15–24 years	2,468	95	26	77,617
25–34 years	10,458	251	35	163,789
35–44 years	26,230	404	42	242,452
45–54 years	63,357	853	65	431,321
55–64 years	138,812	1,884	74	976,021
65–74 years	216,564	2,277	95	1,491,424
75–84 years	243,207	2,327	100	1,767,228
85+ years	242,961	2,196	110	2,087,726
Total	944,650	10,462	90	7,297,815

Source: CDC. (2023, November 9). Provisional death counts for influenza, pneumonia, and COVID-19. https://data.cdc.gov/NCHS/Provisional-Death-Counts-for-Influenza-Pneumonia-a/ynw2-4viq.

from influenza. This represents a ratio of nearly 100:1 in terms of the number of COVID-associated deaths versus influenza deaths. Yet this ratio of deaths is not constant across all ages. A number of observations are salient. First, newborns and infants had a nearly 10-fold higher risk of dying from COVID than influenza. This risk then decreased, both in terms of a relative risk and even in terms of the absolute risk between the ages of 1–14. Children in these age groups had a slightly higher overall risk of dying from COVID than from influenza. Next, both the overall number of fatalities and the ratio of risk of dying went up rapidly with age, particularly in groups aged 75 and above. For individuals 75+, the risk of dying from COVID-19 was approximately 100-fold higher than that of influenza. The elderly are by far the most vulnerable to severe infection, hospitalization, and death.

Again, simply put: COVID-19 was not and is not "just another flu."[55]

Any such demographic table comes with limitations. It condenses lives, stories, meaning, and loss into actuarial tables. We must look at them and grapple with them if we are to respond effectively, while keeping in mind that such statistics do not capture the consequences of a life-changing illness that takes away one's grandparent, parent, sibling, or even child. Yet, by putting these tables together, it helps reinforce the fundamentally different scopes of impact and, ideally, should compel us to react appropriately.

In comparing the deaths caused by COVID-19 with those caused by influenza, we might even consider a hypothetical alternative: a version of the pandemic in which approximately the same number of individuals died of COVID-19 as died of influenza. If that were the case, there would still be twice as many fatalities due to an emerging infectious disease without a vaccine or effective treatment—even this type of threat warrants large-scale public health responses. Instead, this grim statistical table makes it more evident both how much worse COVID-19 was than typical seasonal flu—particularly to the unvaccinated—but also how much of an impact COVID had with respect to the overall risk of dying.

During the 2020–2022 period, COVID-19 became one of the leading causes of mortality across all age groups. For those age 65 and older, the top-three causes of death were heart disease, cancer, and then COVID-19.[56] The risk of dying is much lower in younger age groups, but we should be able to grapple with both facets of this reality without resorting to false dichotomies. By any measure, COVID-19 has been a catastrophe. More than 1 million individuals died in the United States as a result of COVID-19 within two years and a few months after the first documented case, and even this is likely an underestimate of the true burden of mortality in the United States.[57,58] There were approximately 7 million documented fatalities globally as of spring 2023.[59] This number is likely a severe underestimate of the true burden, given the absence of testing, reporting, and documentation in many low- and middle-income countries[60,61] and in China.[62] Yet, it is also true that the increase in the risk of dying is vastly different across ages. For example, what fraction of "excess" deaths are attributable to COVID as a function of age?

Table 1.2 calculates the fraction of total fatalities by age attributable to COVID-19. As is apparent, for the very young, a relatively small fraction (<2.5% for those under age 14) of deaths were likely caused by COVID-19, with this ratio increasing to levels of approximately 1 in 6 for older individuals. And herein lies the tension.

Table 1.2. Relative risk of deaths by age due to COVID-19 (2020–2022)

Age	<1	1–4	5–14	15–24	25–34	35–44	45–54	55–64	65–74	75–84	85+
COVID deaths	0.6%	1.4%	2.3%	3.3%	6.8%	12%	17%	17%	17%	16%	13%

Source: CDC. (2023, November 9). Provisional death counts for influenza, pneumonia, and COVID-19. https://data.cdc.gov/NCHS/Provisional-Death-Counts-for-Influenza-Pneumonia-a/ynw2-4viq.

For someone predisposed to think of COVID-19 as relatively harmless, this table of values could be interpreted to mean that COVID-19 is simply part of life—there are still many other ways to die. Yet, if we ask the same question of heart disease or cancer, would that same COVID skeptic say that we should not make an effort to improve coronary health? Should we stop trying to save lives of those with heart attacks, and should we not try to develop and deploy life-saving cancer treatments? Of course not. That premise is frankly insane—and we can and should reject it. But it is also true that a singular focus on COVID-19 neglects the many ways in which individuals get sick (and die), and that any decision on response that neglects socioeconomic as well as other types of health costs will, over time, be an insufficient and perhaps even the wrong response. It is precisely for this reason that these tables contain, hidden within them, another set of tragedies.

The deaths recorded in table 1.2 span a two-year period. In 2020 and in early 2021, COVID-19 spread throughout the United States among immunologically naive individuals in the absence of large-scale availability of any form of effective drug treatment or vaccine. Age remained the most important driver of differences. Yet age was not the only influential factor linked to the severity of disease and the risk of dying. The risk of dying was also linked to race, ethnicity, and socioeconomic status.

In the first year of the pandemic, the best way to avoid being infected was to limit contacts. Asymptomatic spread meant that a commute, place of work, school, or even family visit could lead to new transmission, even if those around you felt fine. Individuals with white-collar jobs and with greater financial stability, flexibility, and access to paid sick leave were more likely to be able to work from home. Those with greater financial resources were also more likely to be able to secure childcare with better access to testing and infection control. Although people from all walks of life were at risk, there was an obvious and clear relationship between risk and socioeconomic status. Those with fewer financial resources were more likely to have to take public transportation, to work in crowded environments (e.g., in food service, as health care technicians, or in retail or factory settings). Collectively, these exposures increase risk of infection and, ultimately, severe infection and fatalities.[63]

The data provides a context for assessing the relative risk of fatalities across ages during the spread of COVID-19 from early 2020 to early 2022. The link between symptomatic infections and age also cascaded into similar age-specific risks for severe disease, hospitalization, and death. During this two-year period, COVID-19 caused ~100-fold as many fatalities in total as influenza. But during this two-year period, the changes in our behavior also led to fundamental changes in the flu's characteristic annual dynamics. Rather than having intensive spread in the winter, the magnitude of spread was reduced throughout the year. As a result, comparisons of the impact of COVID and influenza might be better put in perspective when taking a "typical" influenza year and asking: To what extent have COVID deaths affected us on an annual basis compared to the expected toll from influenza? Table 1.3 provides an answer.

Table 1.3. Death risk ratio for aggregate COVID-19 fatalities per year (averaged over 2020–2022) vs. influenza deaths (2018–2019)

Age Group	COVID Deaths	Influenza Deaths	COVID:Influenza Death Risk Ratio
<4 years	160	220	~0.72
5–17 years	170	160	~1.1
18–49 years	32,000	1,600	~20
50–64 years	89,000	4,400	~20
65+	350,000	21,000	~17
Total	~470,000	~27,000	~17

Source of flu data: CDC. (2023, August 18, archived). Estimated flu-related illnesses, medical visits, hospitalizations, and deaths in the United States—2018–2019 flu season. https://archive.cdc.gov/#/details?url=https://www.cdc.gov/flu/about/burden/2018-2019.html.

The table compares averaged COVID-19 deaths on an annual basis, grouped by five distinct age groups: those age 4 and younger (including newborns, infants, and small children), children aged 5–17, young and middle-aged adults (aged 18–49), older adults (50–64), and older adults and the elderly (65 and older). Although influenza caused approximately 5,000 fatalities per year since the start of the COVID pandemic, flu typically leads to approximately 25,000 fatalities per year—in that sense the 2018–2019 season is a more appropriate basis for comparison. That is to say that even the comment that COVID-19 "is just flu" misses the reality of the impact that flu has, particularly on the elderly, on an annual basis. Nonetheless, by comparing COVID to a typical flu season, one can see that there is little to no statistical difference in the number of COVID-19 fatalities in children relative to influenza fatalities in children. In every other age group, the risk of dying goes up rapidly and is approximately 20-fold higher than the risk of dying from flu. Once again—rather than thinking about population averages, it is critical to recognize that CO-VID-19 is a very different class of illness than is seasonal influenza, one whose risk to the unvaccinated rises rapidly with age.

It is critical that we face facts regarding COVID-19's impact across ages since its emergence and spread in early 2020:

- Hundreds of children have died of COVID-19 annually in the United States.
- Over 1 million adults have died in total, the vast majority age 65 and older.
- Levels of documented fatalities for children are similar to that of flu.
- Levels of documented fatalities for adults are significantly higher than that of flu, approximately 20-fold higher than in a typical flu season.
- Globally, over 10,000,000 children have lost parents or caregivers due to COVID-19.[64]

The public does not unanimously agree on how to react to these facts, particularly the risks for children and the costs involved in trying to protect them. But we must try to grapple with these facts if we are to bridge the divide and avoid arguing between false dichotomies.

First, COVID-19 is not "just flu." Second, "just flu" is bad, and adding another "just flu" would lead to tens of thousands of new fatalities yearly. Third, many of the same steps that can be taken to reduce COVID-19 infection and fatalities can also reduce the spread and impact of flu. Fourth, the fact that we do not close schools for the flu (except in highly unusual circumstances) raises the question of how best to deal with an illness that has a comparable impact on children (in terms of mortality) as does flu, even if the full spectrum of impacts, including immunological syndromes and other long-term consequences, remains only partially understood. Fifth, even if many (if not most) COVID-19 infections in children caused by existing variants will be mild, some will be severe, others will lead to hospitalizations, and hundreds have been fatal. Finally, the extent of COVID-associated fatalities unfolded despite mitigation measures, like lockdowns and mask mandates, not used against seasonal influenza.

Societies already take significant steps to protect children from mumps, measles, and many other childhood diseases that would—in the past—regularly spread in children, leading to physical injury (scarring), neurological injury (paralysis of movement with polio), and death. It is possible to look at the comparison of COVID-19 and flu deaths by age and suggest that we should have reopened schools by summer 2020 and stopped efforts at control among young children. The data makes it clear that such a choice comes with direct and indirect costs.

In early 2020, Ioannidis and colleagues erroneously claimed that asymptomatic spread was so rampant that COVID-19 was no worse than flu or perhaps even more benign. They were wrong. Yet, we must also avoid paternalism when considering public health policies that affect families who face a spectrum of risks: being one rent check away from homelessness, facing dwindling savings because of pandemic-induced job losses while balancing isolation, health care payments, job insecurity, food insecurity, and worse.

Later in this book we will assess ways that risks of infection and fatalities due to either COVID-19 or flu can be reduced, both for children and for adults. Part of any such strategy must recognize that risk changes with age. The asymptomatic incidence in the young suggests that efforts to prevent spread and the low risk of a fatal outcome must not wait until we find a cluster of symptomatic or severe cases. By then it will be too late—the disease will likely have spread to those far more vulnerable to severe outcomes. But, if we are to drill down into what makes COVID-19 worse than the flu, we must grapple with ways in which the pandemic did not affect everyone equally—especially the gap between mild and severe outcomes.

CHAPTER 2

Mild Cases and Experiential Bubbles

Signals of Airborne Spread

COVID-19 has not been monolithic. Differences in experience and perception are rooted in the core premise of a flawed argument: that asymptomatic infections vastly outnumber symptomatic infections. The mere fact that many individuals had asymptomatic infections left the door open for an alternative narrative to spread—that COVID-19 was not a threat. Asymptomatic and mild infections were in fact common, and they became even more common in the young. But just because someone has an asymptomatic infection does not mean there are no consequences. Someone with a mild or asymptomatic infection can still spread the infection to others, and for them, the outcome could be severe. How can an asymptomatic individual spread a disease to others? Unpacking this question requires thinking about ways that respiratory diseases usually transmit from one person to another and the ways in which COVID-19 may be different.

Typically, we associate an infection with symptoms. And, the telltale symptoms vary with disease type. The common cold is usually accompanied by sneezes, coughs, and a runny nose. Influenza usually brings coughs and a runny nose as well as aches, pains, and a stronger sense of being unwell (to say nothing of those individuals who have sufficiently severe cases that require hospitalization). As such, it seems natural, even intuitive, to attribute the risk of exposing others to the onset of a definitive symptom.

Not only do we typically think of diseases as being transmitted as a result of symptoms, the very symptoms and associated modes of transmission also suggest ways to reduce the risk of infection. If, for example, viruses are spread through mucus, this reinforces the need for increased handwashing. Multiple studies have shown that individuals will increase their frequency of handwashing if they perceive that handwashing is an effective method to stop severe disease.[1] Likewise, if a virus transmits typically through a cough or sneeze, then it reinforces the need to cover one's mouth while coughing and to sneeze into a tissue or handkerchief. Signs posted everywhere from airports to restaurant bathrooms reinforce these commonsense health practices. But how does one try to stop a disease that can be transmitted without symptoms? And perhaps even more challenging, what do we mean by "symptoms" in the first place?

The answer to this question lies in rethinking the ways in which potentially infectious droplets leave the lungs and enter the air. The answer also points to a critical failure of public health agencies—including the World Health Organization (WHO) and the Centers for Disease Control and Prevention (CDC)—to recognize and communicate that which was apparent from early 2020. COVID-19 is and was an airborne disease.

COVID-19 is airborne in the colloquial sense that people understand the term *airborne* to mean that infectious virus particles can spread "through the air." It is also airborne in the sense that very small particles can be released in normal breathing as well as in an occasional sneeze that no one would categorize as definitive proof of being sick. These microscopic particles carry viruses as part of warm breath clouds that do not fall to the ground or bounce off plexiglass barriers like pingpong balls. The life of the very small is not intuitive. Precisely because it is difficult to imagine the trajectory of a cloud of respiratory droplets, it is worth turning to those who have developed new methods to look directly at these otherwise invisible airborne paths.

In March 2020, MIT professor Lydia Bourouiba published images using high-speed digital videos to capture the rapid and relatively long-range dispersal of particles from an individual who breathed, coughed, or sneezed (figure 2.1). (Note: if you listen to her talks, you will learn that Bourouiba induced herself to sneeze many times during the production of the videos.[2]) The premise is to use black-screen methods, a powerful light, and a rapid video capture rate exceeding 1,000 frames per second to capture the still life of airborne spread.[3]

These types of visualization techniques had already been available well before the COVID-19 pandemic. Indeed, Bourouiba and collaborators had been investigating respiratory emissions using a range of visualization and modeling approaches since 2014 with the goal of improving public health and health policy.[4,5] The imaging of the spread of respiratory clouds made it self-evident that a "safe" zone of 3 feet or even 6 feet was hardly a safe limit. Alone, the smaller droplets would

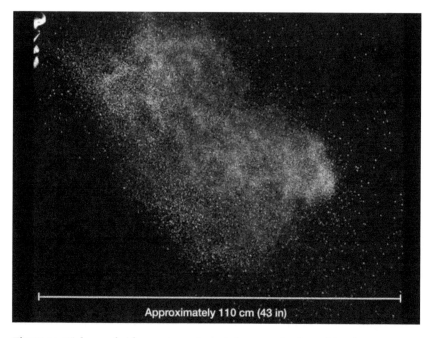

Approximately 110 cm (43 in)

Figure 2.1. High-speed video capture of a turbulent gas cloud resulting from a sneeze. The gas cloud can spread farther than individual droplets—potentially beyond 20 feet. *Source:* Image taken from the work of Lydia Bourouiba (MIT). The image and a full video sequence appear in Bourouiba, L. (2020, March 26). Turbulent gas clouds and respiratory pathogen emissions: Potential implications for reducing transmission of COVID-19. *JAMA* 323: 1837–1838.

rapidly evaporate, and the larger droplets might fall ballistically toward the ground or onto surfaces, unlikely to be inhaled. But respired droplets do not act as singular, ballistic entities. Instead, together, the warm mass of air—a puff—can move together coherently, keeping each droplet protected, and then disperse not just over an initial projectile distance of a few feet but over distances that could travel across an entire room, 20 feet or more.

The fluid dynamics of normal, respiratory air flow implied that waiting for the telltale signs of COVID-19 to initiate preventative steps would almost certainly be a mistake. Transmission did not require characteristic symptoms to release potentially infectious particles in the air. Every breath of an infectious individual could lead to another round of viral release. Small respiratory droplets, spanning the width of a human hair or even 10–100 times smaller, can silently travel across indoor spaces. These particles might even linger in the air well after an infectious person has left. As a result, distance in and of itself is not what mattered but the combination of time, distance, infectiousness, and opportunity.[6,7] And the way to fight back and stop SARS-CoV-2 from getting into the air was to stop individuals from inhaling viruses in the first place—even if no one nearby had a symptom.

In the first few months of 2020, scientists and public health officials suspected that SARS-CoV-2 particles could be transmitted in the air. As but one example, a superspreader event at a Washington State choir practice provided what should have been definitive evidence of airborne spread, spurring public health warnings that physical distancing was not enough to stop transmission.

The Skagit Valley Chorale Superspreading Event

On the evening of March 10, 2020, the Skagit Valley Chorale in Washington State held a rehearsal. This moment of community rapidly became an archetypal example of how hard it would be to stop COVID-19. At the time of the rehearsal, Skagit County had no documented cases, despite increasing reports of illness in the Seattle area. Individuals at the rehearsal were reported to have taken extra precautions, which included not touching one another on arrival and physically distancing in the rehearsal space. The rehearsal lasted multiple hours, indoors, the room filled with song. The act of singing does many things to the singer and the listener. But in the case of a respiratory illness, singing has the unintentional consequence of increasing the dispersal of aerosolized droplets that can spread in the air—and not just over a few feet but across an entire room. That evening, someone in the room was infected (perhaps even more than one person), and they unwittingly sparked a superspreading event. A few days after the rehearsal, multiple individuals reported feeling ill with pneumonia-like symptoms; follow-up tests a week later confirmed the infection was caused by SARS-CoV-2. Ultimately, 53 of the 61 individuals who attended the rehearsal were infected, leading to the deaths of two members of the singing group.[8] One case had become far too many. This pattern of silent spread propagated outward in ever-expanding waves. By April 1, 2020, there were ~200,000 documented cases and more than 5,000 fatalities in the United States,[9] and most of the country was under stay-at-home orders. Despite the obvious severity and need to act, there was paradoxically little actionable information for individuals to take steps to protect their own health and that of their community.

The lesson of the Skagit Valley Chorale was simple and repeated elsewhere (including other super-spreading events globally): one could not simply assume that transmission was linked to definitive symptoms. Instead, individuals who felt (mostly) fine could nonetheless disperse virus particles into the air and infect many others—far too many—without ever feeling that they were sick. So, in any meaningful sense, it was apparent from the beginning that COVID-19 was airborne and that stopping transmission from asymptomatic individuals was going to be critical—because such individuals could release airborne virus particles. Yet, the CDC did not agree. Neither did the World Health Organization (WHO). In fact, both organizations did more than downplay the importance of airborne transmission relative to that of short-distance and even surface-mediated transmission. Instead, both organizations adopted a messaging approach that undermined the notion that COVID-19 could be transmitted in the air.[10]

Charitably, perhaps, the disavowal of COVID-19 airborne transmission reflects the technical expertise of public health professionals and less about the pathogen per se.[11] But it also means that public health organizations were talking to themselves—expert to expert—and not talking to the communities they are meant to serve. For someone working in public health, it is quite important to distinguish, in technical terms, the extent to which a respiratory pathogen is primarily transmitted as either (i) large droplets that fall to surfaces, (ii) small respiratory droplets that can linger in the air before falling (but can infect those approximately 3 feet away), or (iii) smaller aerosolized particles (akin to fine mist) that can linger in the air for minutes or even up to an hour and travel much larger distances. Technically speaking, only the last of these would, in expert terms, be called "airborne transmission." This term is used in the case of measles,[12] but it is not used conventionally for another respiratory disease: influenza. Yet, for the public, any of these three transmission routes are in fact airborne in the sense of being transmitted through the air. Moreover, for COVID-19, there was in fact evidence that droplets were not transmitted ballistically but through airborne mechanisms both in the technical and colloquial sense.

Rather than saying that COVID-19 was airborne, the CDC and WHO declared the opposite. In a moment that did incredible harm and easily could have been avoided, the WHO imprinted its take on public perception as part of a March 28, 2020, tweet that was retweeted nearly 40,000 times (and was covered by press outlets nationally and internationally):[13]

"FACT: #COVID19 is NOT airborne."

This blunt statement was accompanied by a graphic that overlaid the word "INCORRECT" in all capitals and red letters over the phrase "COVID-19 IS CONFIRMED AS AIRBORNE." The fact-check message put the WHO's scientific take in blunt terms: "These droplets are too heavy to hang in the air. They quickly fall on floors or surfaces." In other words, COVID-19 is not airborne.

The consequences of this message cascaded through the public and in public health circles. If COVID-19 was not airborne and the primary route was close contact through droplets, then the priority for preventing transmission should be handwashing, surface cleaning, and avoiding close contact. First, individuals should remain separated, at least 3 feet apart, if not 6 feet for an additional buffer. This would prevent the chance that a respiratory droplet would be directly released and come into contact with the hands, face, and nasal passages of a susceptible individual. Second, surfaces should be cleaned regularly (indeed, many people began wiping down their packages or groceries) because the accumulation of droplets on surfaces could lead to a transmission chain from infected person to surface to susceptible person. Third, plexiglass and other barriers should be placed in indoor spaces to prevent the kind of "splash" zone effect from interactions—especially in high-contact environments such as retail outlets, banks, or schools. Fourth, masking was not an imperative because for those who were asymptomatic, masks would have had little effect—and would perhaps reduce the availability of high-quality masks for medical professionals, given the low supply of masks available in the Strategic National Stockpile.[14] All of these efforts distract from high-impact interventions and may even (in the case of plexiglass barriers) do real harm.[15]

The problem was that COVID-19 was airborne in both a colloquial and a technical sense.[16] The colloquial sense was obvious: virus particles are released during exhalations, coughs, and sneezes. These particles travel through the air in microscopic droplets and can infect others. But the technical sense was in fact more subtle. Public health organizations had historically used a size cutoff of ~5 micrometers as the limiting size below which transmission could be considered airborne.[17] The idea was that large particles would fall to the ground in a matter of seconds and be unlikely to infect others, as long as no one else was in direct contact (e.g., <3 feet away). Yet, as Lydia Bourouiba's videos illustrate, gas clouds of respiratory droplets are comprised of a range of particle sizes. Alone, individual droplets might fall to the ground "ballistically." Surprisingly, these clouds of droplets behave very differently.

The science had indeed evolved, but the response had not.[18]

Bourouiba had shown that a cloud of respiratory droplets protects itself from falling. Warm air rises, and the density of wet, warmer air prevents evaporation while also allowing coherent movement across a room. Imagine the trace of smoke moving in the air from the puff of a cigarette. The telltale sign of smoking can spread throughout a room and linger even after the smoker has departed. The visual and scent signatures of smoke moving through the air are the right analogy for how we should think of the spread of small respiratory droplets. COVID-19 can move invisibly in the air via droplets, not just a few inches or a few feet but potentially dozens of feet across indoor spaces, lingering in the air even after an infectious person has left the room—just like in the case of a smoker's trail. Hence, it is not necessarily proximity that fundamentally matters but whether or not someone has been in a room where someone else with COVID-19 has been breathing, sneezing, or coughing recently. This also means that for all the effort and emphasis on physical distancing, surface cleaning, and plexiglass barriers, the priority should have been elsewhere. And Bourouiba was hardly alone. The story of how a diverse group of scientists from across the globe tried to transform the indoor air landscape is what we consider next.

The Battle for Healthier Air

Indoor air quality science is not necessarily the stuff of popular imagination. The flow of air in homes, schools, shops, or offices seems to lack the broad public interest of topics like dinosaurs, consciousness, and the origin of the universe or life. Yet the science of the built environment is booming—spanning new conferences,[19,20] specialized journals,[21] funding opportunities,[22] and an increasing interest in the consequences of socializing, working, cooking, and sleeping indoors.[23] The Environmental Protection Agency estimates that Americans spend 90% of their time indoors.[24] For respiratory diseases, time spent indoors is precisely the opportunity where transmission is most likely. As such, many experts studying indoor air quality—including scientists across the United States and worldwide such as Kimberly Prather, Linsey Marr,

Lidia Morawska, Joseph Allen, Donald Milton, and others—were prepared to make the case in early 2020 that any substantive response to COVID-19 required a dramatic change in messaging and public health practice. If COVID-19 was airborne—as early indications suggested it most certainly was—then stopping indoor spread must involve a combination of awareness and responses including masks, ventilation, and indoor air filtering. Each plays a complementary role in stopping spread.

Masks help prevent the release of infectious particles into the environment in the first place. Masks can also help a susceptible person avoid infection. Of course, not all masks are equivalent, and their efficacy spans a spectrum from meshed cloth to single-ply masks, three-ply cotton masks, surgical masks, and finally N95-quality masks.[25] Masks also have to be used in the right way and kept on when indoors—not some of the time, but all of the time. When done so, they can reduce the exhalation and inhalation of infectious virus found in respiratory droplets across a range of sizes typically found in gas clouds and, in turn, reduce transmission at population levels.[26] For that same reason, indoor air filters and upper room UV light may also be particularly effective at reducing the risk of transmission (these approaches will be addressed in part 2 of this book).

Next, ventilation is simple—in concept. An open window exchanges air from outside with air inside. The outside air typically has negligibly small levels of virus particles. As such, mixing outdoor air with indoor air dilutes the concentration of virus particles—naturally. The objective, as Kimberly Prather put it, is that "you want the air in your house [or indoors] to be as fresh as the outdoor air."[27]

Air exchange rates dictate just how "fresh" indoor air can be. Imagine there were only one air exchange per hour in an office setting. If so, what fraction of the air molecules would still be present one hour later? The process of exchanging air is random; some molecules move out while new molecules move in. Assuming a random process of exchange leads us to the mathematics of exponentials, instead of growing over time, the chance that the same air is present declines exponentially with time. Technically, approximately e^{-1} of the air moves out after one hour, assuming a rate of one air exchange per hour. That is equivalent to 37% of the air removed, implying that 63% of the air still remains, even with a single air exchange in one hour. Ventilation rates matter, and they have nonlinear and strong impacts on air quality. Imagine increasing ventilation rates to 5 air exchanges per hour. In that case, only e^{-5} of the air remains, or 0.7%, implying that more than 99% of the air has been exchanged. Finally, if ventilation rates increase to 10 air exchanges per hour, then only e^{-10} of the air remains, implying that more than 99.99% of the air will be new after only a single hour of ventilation. Despite the concerns about meeting in person and all the costs of social and physical distancing, one simple approach to improve air quality has been available (when feasible) since the start of the pandemic: outdoor gatherings, open windows, and improved ventilation.

Yet, in many cases, moving outdoors or even opening windows is not feasible. In that case, the principal of indoor air filtration is to cycle air through a filter that reduces the presence of particles, including those as small as a micron in size. In other words, the air continues to move through the room, but with fewer and fewer droplets. These indoor air filters (or scrubbers) work by sending air through a sequence of tiny pores that are large enough for oxygen and carbon dioxide to pass through but too small for the vast majority of respiratory droplets to pass through.[28] These respiratory droplets are removed rapidly from the environment, decreasing the chance that an individual might accidentally inhale an infectious droplet. Fundamentally, the more air exchanges the better, because this progressively (and exponentially) reduces the density of potentially infectious respiratory droplets. The bulk of such droplets are easily filtered out by standard filters (e.g., in the range of a few microns in size). In contrast, SARS-CoV-2 virus particles are on the order of 1/10th of a micron in diameter. This is incredibly small. A human hair is approximately 100 microns in width—equivalent to 1,000 times larger than the width of a single virus particle. On their own, viral particles might be able to pass through mask filters. But virus particles floating in the air are not, in and of themselves, the central danger to infection. Instead, clusters of virus particles are joined in small droplets, and these droplets are precisely the target for air filters. This need not be complex technology. But the state of indoor air—just like the state of water quality—is almost invariably neglected in dense indoor environments. And yet, if we knew (and know) that COVID-19 is airborne and that asymptomatic people can shed infectious viruses even without symptoms, then the priorities for prevention must include efforts to clean the air we breathe indoors.[29]

In early May 2021, the CDC finally updated its guidance on airborne spread. The CDC clarified that the first of the three principal ways by which COVID-19 could spread is through the "inhalation of very fine respiratory droplets and aerosol particles."[30] The right way to interpret this statement is that the inclusion of "very fine respiratory droplets" is a concession to the expansion of the size range of infectious particles that can transmit through the air, potentially at long distances, even if they are not (technically speaking) aerosolized. But the damage had been done. This damage was caused by unnecessary mask wars that were driven in part by confusion, in part by public health guidance, and in part by misinformation that had already become entrenched.[31] In early May 2021, the WHO also declared that COVID-19 was potentially airborne—more than a year too late.

In summary, efforts by the CDC and WHO to readjust policy in line with the scientific evidence (even if contrary to their initial policy declarations) came far too late after already having caused significant harm.

For months, researchers with expertise in the physics of particle and droplet flow (like Lydia Bourouiba[32] and Lidia Morawska[33]), airborne transmission in buildings (like Joseph Allen[34] and Donald Milton[35]), and infection via bioaerosols (like Linsey Marr,[36] Kimberly Prather, Chia Wang, and Robert Schooley[37]) had raised the alarm individually and collectively. In doing so, an entire community of experts working on the problem of airborne transmission had tried to steer the ship of large public health agencies from the outside. For example, in July 2020, more than 200 scientists from across the globe (led by Morawska and Milton) joined together to urge the medical and public health communities to recognize the airborne potential for transmission and revise guidance accordingly. Their central scientific conclusion was straightforward:

Studies by the signatories and other scientists have demonstrated beyond any reasonable doubt that viruses are released during exhalation, talking, and coughing in microdroplets small enough to remain aloft in air and pose a risk of exposure at distances *beyond* 1–2 m from an infected individual.[38]

The key term "beyond" is italicized here for emphasis. But the other key terms are the modalities by which COVID-19 can spread, including exhalation, talking, and coughing. Exhalation and talking are obviously not a telltale sign of infection.

This statement and the wide range of evidence that supported it were present in public discourse from the earliest moments, and they were often the subject of the CDC's investigative reports. The choir incident in Washington State ended up being one of such reports.[39] The Skagit Valley Chorale superspreading event was an early example of the potential that one case could become many, even if an infectious individual felt fine. Given the intensity of spread, the follow-up investigation formed the centerpiece of an analysis on a "high attack rate" at a choir practice published on May 15, 2020, in the CDC's most prestigious in-house publication: *Morbidity and Mortality Weekly Report*.[40] Colloquially referred to as the *MMWR*, this publication is known as the "the voice of CDC."[41] The choir practice article speculated on transmission modalities, including the possibility that there was something special about singing and its potential to increase aerosolization. Yet the search for unusual circumstances associated with superspreading overlooked the banal and the obvious: COVID-19 was in fact airborne.

One additional example is shown below. It depicts a chain of transmission of COVID-19 as a result of long-distance infection at a restaurant in Guangzhou, China. Guangzhou is a megacity in Southern China, less than 100 miles as the crow flies from Hong Kong. On January 24, 2020, a family who had been in Wuhan Province traveled to Guangzhou and went for lunch. Multiple other diners were present. Within days, individuals from the other families became sick—rapid PCR (polymerase chain reaction) tests identified the cause as SARS-CoV-2. The infected individual had sat more than 3 feet away from those who would become infected. The investigative team ruled out the potential that staff were infected or the air conditioner in the restaurant had somehow been contaminated. The investigative team also ruled out other potential infectious contacts among the two family groups that were affected. Instead, the parsimonious explanation is that one individual from family group "A" infected multiple other family groups (potentially causing secondary infection chains in those families). As is apparent, the distance from the primary case to two of the other cases is more than 10 feet. The investigative report was published in the CDC's journal *Emerging Infectious Disease*, and although the official publication date was July 2020, the article was released online in April 2020. The author team downplayed the possibility that droplets could have stayed in the air long enough to infect other groups; instead they attributed the long-distance transmission to the additional flow of air (both the outlet and return of air were located above table C in figure 2.2).

As in the Washington State choir case, the conventional assumption that droplets rapidly fall out of the air led public health organizations to seek special explanations for "long distance" spread. These special explanations included aerosolization of viruses during singing, the particular speed/orientation of air-conditioning units, or the possibility that some individuals are "super-emitters" of high infectious loads of virus particles. Each of these mechanisms may be at play. Unfortunately, special explanations are not required.

The parsimonious explanation for the choir practice and other superspreading events is, unfortunately, more mundane. Individuals who are infected can release enough infectious viral particles in small respiratory droplets that stay aloft, spread in the air, and infect others. Moreover, individuals need not have symptoms—or ever exhibit clinical symptoms—to infect others. The evidence for asymptomatic and airborne spread was present from near the beginning of the pandemic, even if conventional theory disregarded such spread as a major mechanism for transmission. This is what new evidence is for: it helps scientists revise and extend understanding as part of an iterative process. Such iteration is at the core of the scientific method. Yet, not only does asymptomatic transmission help spread COVID-19, but its existence

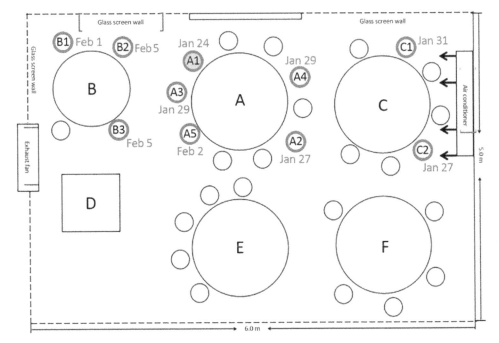

Figure 2.2. Sketch of the transmission from an index case (gray circle denoted as A1) to new cases (open circles) at a restaurant in Guangzhou Province, China. Distinct family groups are denoted by the letters A, B, and C. The room dimensions are 6 meters × 5 meters. *Source*: Reproduced in grayscale from the figure in Lu, J., et al. (2020). COVID-19 outbreak associated with air-conditioning in restaurant, Guangzhou, China, 2020. *Emerging Infectious Diseases* 26: 1628–1631. https://doi.org/10.3201/eid2607.200764. Licensed under Creative Commons BY 4.0 DEED, Attribution 4.0 International. https://creativecommons.org/licenses/by/4.0/.

also underlies a perceptual difference. The chance that someone can be infected and have a mild or asymptomatic case changes rapidly with age.

Age and Asymptomatic Infections

It is hard to fight an unseen enemy. Asymptomatic spread means that individuals can infect others even when they seem to feel fine. But the chances of asymptomatic spread are not constant from person to person, and they are certainly not constant across different groups of people. Perhaps the cumulative epidemic impact and our collective reactions to the threat of COVID-19 might have been different if we all—in some fundamental sense—felt we were in the fight together.

Of course, we are linked—from the perspective of disease transmission—irrespective of how we might feel about risk. What happens in one household, one place of work, or one social event rarely stays there. The virus spreads from person to person and from one to many, but in doing so, the experience of COVID-19 is vastly different. This is where the fight and experience differs.

The accumulation of case studies and models helped build an evidence base in early to mid-2020 that approximately half of COVID-19 infections lead to mild/asymptomatic outcomes.[42] This is a population-level average. It does not mean that one-half of young people and one-half of older people will have an asymptomatic infection. To the contrary, the chances of asymptomatic outcomes depend on numerous cofactors and potentially even the context in which one is exposed. Yet, despite all the efforts to identify those factors that differentiated those who became severely ill from those who ended up with mild or even asymptomatic infections, one factor was and has remained the most important, the most evident, and the most likely to drive outcome.

That factor is age.

The young, including children, teenagers, and young adults (18 to 34 years old) are significantly more likely to have a mild or asymptomatic infection and therefore significantly less likely to end up hospitalized or admitted to the intensive care unit (ICU) when compared to middle-aged individuals (35 to 59 years old). Yet, children and teenagers tend to have high contact rates in school settings,[43] and young adults have about the highest levels of mobility of any age group.[44] This means there can be a gap between their personal risk and their potential for transmission. Although the risk of severe outcomes increases with age, middle-aged individuals are significantly less likely to have a severe outcome when compared to older individuals (e.g., those age 60+), and therefore they are significantly less likely to end up hospitalized or in the ICU. Individuals 60 years of age and older are at a higher risk of having a symptomatic and potentially a severe case on average, with risks rising even faster for those age 70 or above and even more so for those age 80 and above. The relationship between age and severity transcends national boundaries. But it is worthwhile to explore one of the earliest examples to illustrate how rapidly it became apparent that outcome was linked to age.

Figure 2.3 highlights differences in symptomatic and critical illness across different age groups. The data comes from the Lombardy region in Italy and focuses on individuals who had a close contact with a confirmed COVID-19 case. The observations were collected from February to April 2020, at the moment when Lombardy and Northern Italy were hit hard by SARS-CoV-2.

The study revealed differences in outcomes between females (left) and males (right), with males tending to exhibit more severe outcomes in each age group. What should be even more apparent is that approximately 1 in 5 cases of individuals 80 years of age or older ends up requiring critical care. In contrast, none of the observed cases in this particular study for those age 20 and younger required critical care. Such

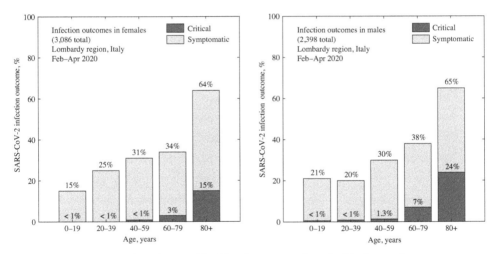

Figure 2.3. Age- and gender-specific risk of symptomatic and critical cases for females (left panel) and males (right panel) from a study in Lombardy, Italy, of COVID-19 cases identified between February 21, 2020, and April 16, 2020. *Source*: Redrawn with data from the figure in Poletti, P., et al. (2021). Association of age with likelihood of developing symptoms and critical disease among close contacts exposed to patients with confirmed SARS-CoV-2 infection in Italy. *JAMA Network Open* 4: e211085. https://doi.org/10.1001/jamanetworkopen.2021.1085.

initial results must be placed into context—for example, if enough infections happen, then the odds increase that some children, teenagers, and young adults may have severe outcomes or even die of the disease. These are tragedies—tragedies compounded when there is a failure to control the overall rate of spread. Eventually, even with a small percentage of severe outcomes, the odds catch up. But, the primary message should also resonate. The nature of COVID-19 is fundamentally different between the young and the old. As the authors noted:

> In this Italian cohort study of close contacts of patients with confirmed SARS-CoV-2 infection, more than one-half of the individuals tested positive for the virus. However, most infected individuals did not develop respiratory symptoms or fever.[45]

This shift in age-dependent outcomes immediately suggests two key consequences for awareness, spread, and control.

First, if we want to understand what might happen as COVID-19 spreads across a population, then we must also consider the age distribution of the population—that is, demographics matters.[46] Consider an outbreak that spreads in a college dorm versus an outbreak that spreads in a long-term care facility. Both may have 200 residents in addition to staff members who work at the facility. But the expected outcomes are markedly different. In the case of the college dorm, if 50% of the residents are infected, then it is quite plausible, if not likely, that none would experience a critical case requiring hospitalization. There will certainly be exceptions, but rapid spread of asymptomatic, mild, and some symptomatic infections would be the norm. The outcome in a long-term care facility could not be more distinct. In the case of a long-term care facility with 200 residents, a large-scale outbreak infecting 50% of residents might lead to dozens of hospitalizations and multiple fatalities.

This comparison separates transmissibility from severity. Indeed, the fraction of individuals infected in a college or a nursing home may be equal, even as the number of severe outcomes is markedly different. Consequently, trying to make sense of large-scale outbreaks requires considering how age differences act as a filter, with cases increasing in severity progressively in a hockey-stick or J-shaped fashion. The older one is, the worse the outcome is likely to be. Therefore, populations with divergent age structures can experience markedly different outbreak outcomes. Groups of young individuals will have far more mild outcomes than groups of older individuals—and both groups will have outcomes that look very different from the overall population average. This difference underlies the second major consequence of the link between age and asymptomatic infections.

Differences in age-dependent outcomes can be compounded by the fact that individuals often socialize with individuals of a similar age. This means that individual experiences and indeed perceptions of the severity of COVID-19 can differ dramatically with age. This kind of within-age socialization is typical. Social interaction studies conclude that there is a strong tendency for individuals to interact with peers of a similar age—an unsurprising result with far-reaching consequences.[47] Colleges and long-term care facilities represent somewhat extreme examples. In both cases, individuals within each facility are more similar in age than would typically be the case for two random individuals from the population at large. As a consequence, a 20-year-old in a dorm is far more likely to spend time with another 20-year-old (or an 18- or 22-year-old) than with someone age 40, 50, or 60, particularly indoors in contexts that could potentially lead to spread. Likewise, the gathering of residents for meals in an active retirement community or in a long-term care facility leads to a different kind of age-specific mixing, albeit among older individuals. Inevitably, there will be interactions that go outside these age groups (e.g., the occasional visit of adult children and young grandchildren to a long-term care facility). This "leakage" outside similar age groups can have dramatic consequences. Nonetheless, the tendency for within-age interactions can shape the perception of COVID-19 severity.

On Colleges and Long-Term Care Facilities

Let us expand our examination of COVID-19 spread on a college campus and consider 50 people living in a fraternity that was not designed to provide air isolation between living quarters, restrooms, and eating spaces. In some sense, Greek houses on college campuses (as well as some dormitories and residence halls) are akin to cruise ships at rest: they are vulnerable to rapid spread of airborne and even foodborne infections. But because asymptomatic outcomes are more likely in the young, one can assume that a small fraction (e.g., 1 in 500 for ease of illustration) of unvaccinated and otherwise healthy 20-year-olds will end up hospitalized after a COVID-19 infection. Hospitalization may include a brief visit to be evaluated and discharged, yet even this kind of event can mark a community's perception of severity. Consider what happens if 50% of fraternity house members are infected—a large outbreak. Despite the numbers of infections, we expect no one to be hospitalized in 95% of such outbreaks. If hospitalization rates are closer to 1 in 1,000 and the outbreak leads to 10 infections, then the odds increase to 99% that no one will be hospitalized in the entire outbreak.[48] If one were to ask a member of a fraternity or sorority house what COVID-19 was like during the fall 2020 to spring 2021 semesters, they might conclude that yes, many got infected, but the experience of having COVID-19 was not that bad.

This statement might make some feel uncomfortable. It should. But, go ahead, ask a college student. For them and the bulk of their peers, their personal experience of a COVID-19 infection might have represented a few days of inconvenience. For others, many students may never have realized that they were infected at all due to a combination of mild (or no) symptoms and the inadequacy of testing. Others may have been tested through a campus program, learned they were infected, but had no evident symptoms. Of course, at a societal level, COVID-19 has been a catastrophe. But, if we are to communicate risk as it is, then we should not apply population-level averages to groups with markedly different risk factors. Why should a college student who sees that 25 of their close friends have been infected with either no symptoms, mild symptoms, or a few days of lying in bed believe that the entire world should be turned upside down? If major changes are needed in the way that we organize our live-learn environments, then we should explain the reasons why. We should not exaggerate the risks of fatalities in their age group and misleadingly claim that typical college students are at a high risk of a fatal infection. If leaders do so, then the lived reality and public health messaging will be discordant—undermining trust in the very platforms used to try and control spread.

A thoughtful COVID-19 mitigation and response campaign must be nuanced and recognize the reality of the relatively low risk of severe outcomes in young adults. Collectively, this low risk can lead to realized experiences that can then quickly be shared not just in that one fraternity house or dorm but between friends and peer groups and on social media, reinforcing a dominant paradigm: COVID-19 is not that bad after all; perhaps it is no worse than the flu. If college students are told that "we" are all going to die, then they will tune out such alarmism just as they tune out other peddlers of misinformation. They might even conclude that the "we" referenced in public health campaigns does not necessarily include them. Rather than fatalities per se, the more likely risks for a college student are a longer period of recovery—analogous to post-mono or post-flu recovery but potentially worse—involving chronic fatigue, brain fog, or problems with breathing that affect everything from basic physical activities to sports.[49] These lived risks are substantive and damaging and not what a college students wants to experience.

And yet, college students do not just stay in their dorms.

Let us now revisit the case of a long-term care facility and consider the consequences of an outbreak in a community with 100 residents where one-half of them become infected. In 2020, the risk of hospitalization from a COVID-19 infection for an otherwise healthy 75-year-old was many times higher than for an otherwise healthy 20-year-old. One person in a dozen might require hospitalization at age 75, rather than one person in many hundreds at age 20. These odds can rapidly increase with comorbidities. Together, this means that a severe outbreak in a long-term care facility of 100 residents could lead to 50 cases and a half-dozen hospitalizations (or more, depending on the frailty of the residents). Residents, caregivers, and their families would therefore experience COVID-19 risk in an entirely different way. For them, the default expectation is that COVID-19 is a severe disease. Outbreaks in long-term care facilities would almost certainly involve the recurring sound of ambulances arriving to the site, taking individuals from facilities into hospitals and ICUs—and, unfortunately, many of those admitted would never return. This grim fact is widely understood for anyone whose relatives or loved ones lived in long-term care facilities.

An estimated 1 in 12 individuals who lived in long-term care facilities and 1 in 10 individuals who lived in nursing homes in the United States died of COVID-19 during the first year of the pandemic.[50] In total, nearly 1 in 3 fatalities in the first year of COVID-19 in the United States were among residents of long-term care facilities, despite the fact that residents of these facilities represented 1% of all documented infections—a 30-fold higher risk of fatality per each documented infection.

Age, symptoms, and severity. The link has been clear from the beginning. And yet, precisely because of the massive difference in outcomes, any discussion of COVID-19 outcomes should come with a caveat.

First and foremost: age matters. This is not to discount other issues. There are many ways in which ethnicity, socioeconomic status, gender, comorbidities (particularly those related to respiratory function) affect the risk of symptoms, severity, and fatalities.[51,52] But we must first reconcile how asymptomatic outcomes change markedly with age. If we do not, then we have missed the opportunity to focus on how individuals experiences are likely going to differ. For those who are older, the risk that a COVID-19 infection leads to severe illness is far higher than for a young adult living at college. This difference means we need to talk differently to different groups, emphasizing the difference between infection, symptoms, and transmissibility.

Because what happens in the college dorm does not just remain there. The very same studies that have found that individuals tend to preferentially interact with individuals of the same or similar age also find that such preferential interaction is not universal. People mix. This mixing means that one's perception of what might be acceptable behavior in one age (or risk) group is not necessarily perceived to be acceptable in a different age (or risk) group. Given the increasing risk of severe outcomes with age, there is a risk that mixing between young and older individuals could catalyze spread, albeit unintentionally. Two examples illustrate this point.

The first example involves the movement of college-age students back from their fall or spring semesters, particularly fall semesters, when a return home for Thanksgiving or Christmas breaks usually involves family and multigenerational gatherings. These gatherings almost certainly accelerated the spread of COVID-19 in fall 2020.[53] Students living in dense live-learn environments where COVID-19 was spreading may have been infected asymptomatically, especially given the public health risk posed by the large density and interaction rates on college campuses. Many colleges moved nearly entirely online in spring 2020 and fall 2020. Nonetheless, many colleges welcomed back students into dorms with limited (or no) rapid or next-day viral testing, using a mix of online and in-person formats for instruction. Whereas the perception of COVID-19 might have been shaped by the relatively mild presentation on campuses, a trip home could be fraught. Older individuals who may have spent many months limiting their interactions began to interact with their children or grandchildren who may have unwittingly brought a virus into a family gathering. Given how often college-age individuals had mild or asymptomatic cases, such gatherings could then trigger regret or worse.

The second example involves the care of older (and often frail) individuals in long-term care (LTC) facilities and nursing homes. The staff in such facilities are far too often underpaid and overworked.[54] Staff members are typically significantly younger than the individuals they care for. In many instances, such facilities initiated systemic infection control protocols in an effort to protect vulnerable residents. In aggregate, such efforts failed. Ultimately, the timing of outbreak surges in LTCs coincided with the waxing and waning of cases in the community.[55] One mechanism to explain this link is the potential that staff members were themselves infected during community surges. In essence, the same people who tried to provide care for older residents could become the same people who unwittingly brought the virus into the facility. Caring for older, medically frail individuals is hard work—physically, emotionally, and mentally. It can also be rewarding work. Yet such facilities are hardly bubbles, sealed off from the outside world. The same staff who work day and night to provide care also go to the supermarket and stores and live in households with their own risk factors. The net result is that the interaction of an asymptomatically infected individual can be devastating—not for them, but for those in their orbit.

In short, in the perceptual universe of a child or college student, COVID-19 might be largely a mild or asymptomatic disease. In the perceptual universe of those living in retirement homes or nursing homes, COVID-19 is a severe threat, leading to symptomatic disease and an elevated chance of hospitalization or death. Sustaining measures to stop spread comes with costs. In the United States, the response to COVID-19 was distributed and heterogeneous, leaving states on their own to decide on rules and responses. Indeed, sometimes responses were left to cities to make up for the absence of a coordinated national response.[56] As the buck got passed, more and more folks became confused by changing guidance, different experiences, and deliberate misinformation. Was COVID-19 largely asymptomatic or not? Was it airborne or not? Was it time to wear masks or not? And was it time to let go of stringent restriction or perhaps even to become more cautious as cases and the intensity of spread increased?

The United States is large and complex; some might argue that it is too large for a one-size-fits-all approach, especially given the ethos that many decisions should be left up to individuals and not the state.[57] Taken to extremes, such perspectives can lead to individuals acting in their own self-interest but ending up with worse outcomes than had they coordinated. A tragedy of the commons can arise when individual interests are not aligned with collective interests—and when mutual coercion to enforce social norms are not mutually agreed on. But agreement on how to react to COVID-19 was always going to be hard. Individuals perceived the risk of COVID-19 differently—at some level because risk was truly different and at another level because individuals received (and/or amplified) different types of (mis)information about the realized threat from the pandemic. In the absence of a universal link between symptoms and transmission, individuals often had to make difficult choices constrained by far more than just the risk of being infected.

Symptoms, Severity, and Transmissibility

Ebola virus disease (EVD) is a devastating illness. Individuals infected with EVD almost invariably develop severe symptoms, with fatality rates often exceeding 50%.[58,59] Supportive care can improve outcomes, but a significant fraction of infected individuals eventually die. EVD spreads through direct contact with bodily fluids of an infected individual. Those at greatest risk are often family members, caregivers, and medical staff—anyone who is close enough to try and help. Precisely for this reason, medical teams working with EVD patients wear full protective gear, and ideally, treatment takes place in Ebola treatment units with specialized wards, which reduces risk to caregivers. Such precautions only go so far, as early symptoms of EVD can mimic those of malaria—and medical staff experience higher rates of infection and fatalities than do the population at large. Consider this one grim statistic: approximately 1 in 1,000 of the general population in Liberia died of EVD between March 2014 and May 2015, compared to 1 in 12 of the country's health care workers.[60]

Given the telltale signs of EVD, individuals who experience severe bone aches and hemorrhagic fevers (reaching above 107 degrees) are typically unable to move beyond their bed or home. These individuals continue to shed virus during their symptomatic phase. Precisely because of the severe symptoms, it is possible to develop communication and response strategies that aim to minimize contact with infected individuals and even to minimize contact with the bodies of individuals who have died of EVD. As it turns out, it is possible to contract EVD during the preparation of bodies for burial. [61] The handling and washing of bodies before death is common in many cultures—so too in West Africa. In the event that someone has died of EVD, such funeral practices can put susceptible individuals in direct contact with infectious bodily fluids. For infected individuals, EVD is one of the worst diseases known to humans. Yet even the largest EVD outbreak recorded in 2014–2015 in West Africa caused no more fatalities than does seasonal flu in the United States in a typical year.

Ebola may appear to be an extreme example of a disease in which symptoms are linked to transmission and severe outcomes at the individual level. But SARS-1 is another, and it is perhaps a more relevant example of the gap between individual fatality risk and aggregate population fatalities.

The SARS-1 outbreak emerged in late 2002 in mainland China, about 100 miles north of Hong Kong, before spreading to adjacent regions, including Hong Kong, Vietnam, and Taiwan. SARS-1 is caused by a coronavirus similar to SARS-CoV-2. At the individual level, SARS-1 was more severe than SARS-CoV-2, leading to higher rates of hospitalization and far higher case fatality rates. Early reports estimated a case fatality rate of ~13% for individuals younger than age 60 and ~43% for individuals older than 60,[62] although these rates declined with time. In response, individuals in affected Asia Pacific regions rapidly adopted preventative measures, including mask-wearing and avoiding crowded areas.[63] These measures were complemented by rapid contact tracing and isolation. In total, nearly 800 individuals died of SARS-1 of the approximately 8,000 documented infections. This corresponds to a case fatality rate (CFR) of ~10%. Yet, SARS-1 had a particular feature that made it, like EVD, easier to control at the population level, even as it remained a devastating illness to infected individuals.[64] For SARS-1, the peak levels of viral load occurred multiple days *after* the onset of symptoms,[65] and there was far less evidence of meaningful asymptomatic transmission. Reviewing the epidemiological impacts of SARS-1 in 2004, a group of scientists concluded:

> The low transmissibility of the virus, combined with the onset of peak infectiousness following the onset of clinical symptoms of disease, transpired to make simple public health measures, such as isolating patients and quarantining their contacts, very effective in the control of

the SARS epidemic. We conclude that we were lucky this time round, but may not be so with the next epidemic outbreak of a novel aetiological agent.[66]

We may have been lucky with SARS-1, but we were not lucky with SARS-CoV-2.

On February 23, 2020, a worrisome preprint was posted on MedRxiv—the same electronic sharing mechanism used by John Ioannidis and colleagues to report results from their Santa Clara serological survey. The paper, led by Lauren Ancel Meyers of the University of Texas at Austin and colleagues in France, mainland China, and Hong Kong, focused on the link (or lack thereof) between symptoms and transmissibility.[67] The conventional way to characterize this link is to measure a feature of a disease termed "the serial interval." The serial interval is defined as the time between when a primary case exhibits symptoms and the time that secondary cases exhibit symptoms—in other words, it is the difference between illness onset in the infector and infectee. For SARS-CoV-2, the incubation period was estimated to be 4 to 6 days. If transmission occurred after the onset of symptoms, then one would expect that the serial interval would be centered at a serial interval *exceeding* this incubation period. Moreover, if peak viral load followed the onset of symptoms, then it would be plausible to imagine that the serial interval could be centered at approximately 10 days. Such a gap indicates that an individual was infected, had an incubation period, exhibited symptoms, and then experienced peak infectiousness before recovering.

To explore this in more detail, consider a newly infected individual—the primary case. Imagine that the primary case takes 5 days to exhibit symptoms, arising in part due to viral proliferation and the immune system response. Denote this symptom onset date as day 0. If transmissibility is linked to viral load, and viral load takes 5 days to reach its peak, then most of the infections linked to the primary case will occur approximately on day 5. As a result, newly infected individuals will tend to be infected approximately 5 days after the primary case symptom onset and will themselves take 5 more days to exhibit symptoms—with a mean closer to 10 days. Individual transmission events depend not just on viral load but on interactions. Consequently, epidemiologists tend to group all of these serial intervals together to form a distribution—the serial interval distribution. Figure 2.4 shows this systematic report of the serial interval distribution for COVID-19.

To those accustomed to interpreting serial intervals and chains of transmission, this distribution shown in figure 2.4 was disturbing. Approximately 25% of the transmission events had a zero value or negative serial interval. This corresponds to a situation where the infected individual exhibited symptoms on the same day (or before!) the primary case. One might ask, how is this possible? A zero-value or negative

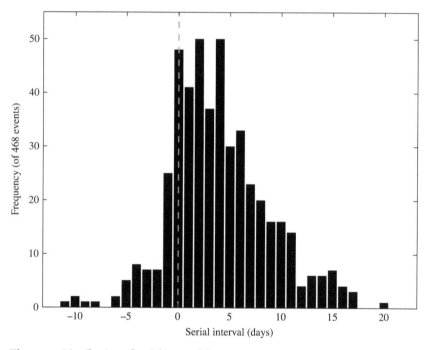

Figure 2.4. Distribution of serial interval from transmission events in China between January 21, 2020, and February 8, 2020. Bars denote the frequency of intervals among the transmission events, and the dashed line corresponds to a serial interval of zero. *Source*: Adapted from data in the preprint Du, Z., et al. (2020, March 20). The serial interval of COVID-19 from publicly reported confirmed cases. MedRxiv. https://doi.org/10.1101/2020.02.19.20025452. Published version (2020) in *Emerging Infectious Diseases* 26: 1341–1343.

serial interval implies that the primary case was infectious presymptomatically and passed on the infection in the absence of clinical symptoms. Moreover, approximately 66% of all transmission events had a serial interval shorter than an incubation period of 5 days. The link between primary and secondary case is difficult and often requires detailed public health investigations—for example, identifying individuals who had contacts with known infected cases. The finding of a significant proportions of negative, zero-valued, or short serial intervals heightens the risk that an emerging infectious disease will be difficult to control.

When symptoms are linked to transmission, then it is possible to leverage symptom identification as a means to take action, especially when such transmission involve close contact. The finding of substantial levels of zero-valued and negative serial intervals in February 2020 only elevated deep concern—SARS-CoV-2 was fundamentally unlike SARS-1. In chapter 3, we go one step further—explicitly incorporating evidence of asymptomatic transmission into principled mechanistic models of disease spread to assess just how and why asymptomatic transmission between individuals can make disease outcomes worse at population scales.

CHAPTER 3

Asymptomatic Transmission Leads to Many More Fatalities

The Infection Begins within a Host

Asymptomatic transmission is a double-edged sword. On the one hand, it would seem that the very existence of asymptomatic cases would be good news. If people can have mild cases, that seems to imply that the disease may be less dangerous to populations as a whole. It turns out this reasoning is flawed. Paradoxically, what is good for an individual can be bad for the population. Why? Because individuals who are asymptomatically *infected* can nonetheless infect others. The double-edge sword is dangerous precisely because asymptomatic infection is good news with respect to the severity of a disease, but asymptomatic *transmission* (i.e., the ability of asymptomatically infected individuals to infect others) can make epidemic outcomes worse.

This seemingly paradoxical idea will take a while to unpack. But, if we are not willing to do so, then we have not taken the necessary steps to understand precisely why the deck was stacked against public health response efforts, why many tried to raise the alarm on asymptomatic infections, and why governments and public health officials (in the United States and in countries worldwide) were unable to effectively stop the spread of COVID-19.

What does asymptomatic transmission even mean, and why is it different from the fact that SARS-CoV-2 can lead to asymptomatic infections?

To begin, consider a healthy adult who is exposed to SARS-CoV-2 somewhere—whether in their family living room, a restaurant, a store, a place of work, a theater, a chorus practice, or a cafe. The exposure takes place because someone in the room is infected and has been shedding viruses, a lungful at a time. Now, the chances that you breath in a virus particle drops dramatically if you are wearing a mask—and, better yet, a high-quality mask (an issue we will return to later). Even if you are not wearing a mask (or even if you are, but have been unlucky because of the mask's quality, fit, or condition), the entry of a virus particle into your lungs does not guarantee you will become infected. As a rule, the more virus particles you inhale, the higher the chance that you will become infected (i.e., the "dose" matters).

The infectious dose represents the estimated number of pathogens typically required to initiate an infection. It can take millions or more of *Vibrio cholerae* cells to initiate a cholera infection in healthy adults.[1] In contrast, it only takes a few dozen cells of the enterohemorrhagic strains of *E. coli* to initiate a potentially fatal infection,[2] which is yet another reason why you should wash vegetables, cook ground beef thoroughly, and watch out for alfalfa sprouts. For SARS-CoV-2, current estimates suggest that it may take only a few hundred virus particles to potentially initiate an infection.[3] This means that if you are standing close to someone who is infected, then the local concentration of virus particles in the air will be higher, and your infection risk will also be higher. Over time, if you keep standing there (without a mask on), the odds increase that one of the virus particles secures a foothold and infects an epithelial cell in your lungs and starts to proliferate.

The risk of infection goes up with time and down with distance, which is also the reason that early interventions and criteria for "close contacts" often refer to the 6 feet and 15 minute rule. Of course, such rules represent an approximation to the reality, particularly in light of airborne transmission (described in chapter 2). The actual risk represents a combination of time, distance, and the level of viral release. These factors are hard to measure simultaneously and represent confusing standards. It is also why indoor dining represents a significantly elevated risk environment for spread. Even if you are sitting more than 6 feet away from the nearest patron, after an hour without a mask, then the virus particles being emitted 10 or even 20 feet away are likely floating in the air, right next to you . . . and in you.

It is also possible that you may breathe in a more concentrated form of virus particles: a respiratory droplet. Respiratory droplets can be a micrometer in dimension. For context, that is about the size of a typical bacteria, or 1/100th the width of a human hair. In contrast, the SARS-CoV-2 virus is approximately 1/10th of a micron in diameter.[4] This means that an exhaled respiratory droplet of about 1 micron in diameter could contain on the order of a thousand (or more) viruses. Hence, a single inhalation event of a respiratory droplet could be enough to initiate an infection. If you are close enough to someone to breathe in a single droplet containing a thousand viruses, then it will not matter that your interactions were incidental—you may already be infected.

The term *infection* is more stringent than that of exposure. Infection means that the virus can replicate inside human cells, turning individual cells into virus factories. Each cell can be filled with large numbers of virus particles at a given moment in time.[5] These viruses can spread to uninfected cells in different ways. First, virus particles can be released from infected cells inside a human host. These virus particles contain the viral genome inside a protective capsid. The human immune system can wipe out virus particles before they find a new cellular home to infect and take over—with virus particle viability assumed to last a few hours.[6] This implies that the introduction of virus particles inside the lungs does not lead, inevitably, to the initiation of infection. But, if infections are initiated, then individual cells can become virus factories, leading to concentrations of tens of thousands of virus particles inside a single infected cell, which can then be released and enter other susceptible cells.[7] Second, viruses can spread directly between cells.[8] This kind of direct link is often harder for the immune system to detect because viruses leverage connections between cells as a way to avoid triggering some of the hallmark systems—including neutralizing antibodies—that the human immune system uses to detect and eliminate pathogens. Either way, the accumulation of infection, production, and reinfection leads to a potentially exponential growth of viruses and infected cells.[9]

Exponentials are fast. They are also hard to fathom—as illustrated in figure 3.1.

The figure shows what would happen if the number of infectious units were to double each "generation" as viruses spread from cell to cells within a human lung. A single infectious unit becomes 128 within 7 generations of infection. Imagine that each generation lasts

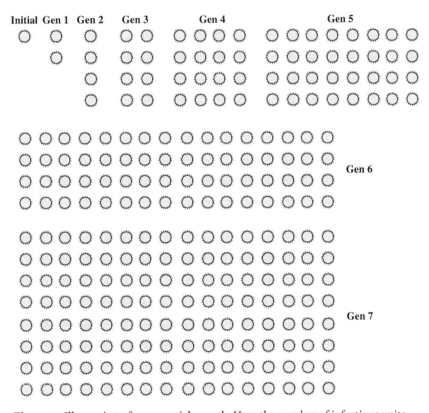

Figure 3.1. Illustration of exponential growth. Here the number of infectious units doubles each cellular generation (Gen). By generation 7, there are more than 100 infectious units; by generation 14, there are more than 16,000 (not shown); and by generation 21, there are more than 2 million (not shown).

approximately six hours. Within 7 generations, there would be more than 16,000 infectious units, and 7 generations later, there would be over 2 million—approaching lower estimates of the total number of target lung cells that SARS-CoV-2 viruses infect.[10] In this example, this means that in ~21 generations—just over five days—a few viruses can lead to a massive lung infection along with symptoms. Symptoms arise from two main sources: the harm that the virus causes to us and the harm that we cause to ourselves as a result of the immune system fighting off the virus.[11]

In summary, an infection progresses through a series of stages, catalyzed by the inhalation of an initially small number of viruses. Some of these virus particles are infectious and bind to target cells in the epithelial layer of the lungs (i.e., the interface between the tissue and the airways). These viruses turn infected cells into virus factories, releasing more viruses that then infect new cells and continue to proliferate. The immune system begins to recognize both infected cells and virus particles and initiates an immune response. If effective, the specific virally infected cells and virus particles are systematically cleared. In good scenarios, the immune system starts to win, the infected cells are killed (even as target cells are depleted by the process of infection, depriving the infection of its force), and soon, the losses (for the virus) are greater than the gain, and the infection dies out, also exponentially fast.

This boom-and-bust cycle may not necessarily lead to something that a clinician would call a symptomatic case. Certainly, if we were to peer into lung tissue or use a PCR (polymerase chain reaction)-based molecular viral test, then we could find evidence of an infection. Yet, operationally, an infected individual may feel fine or have mild or non-specific symptoms that range from a slightly runny nose, the slight feeling of being out of sorts, or perhaps an occasional cough or a mild headache or low-grade fever. None of these symptoms need be associated with SARS-CoV-2. And clinicians do not typically order diagnostic or invasive tests for every sneeze, sniffle, and cough. Infectiousness need not be precisely correlated to symptoms. Indeed, there is ample evidence that asymptomatic individuals can shed nearly as much virus for nearly as long as symptomatically infected individuals (figure 3.2).

National Basketball Association (NBA)

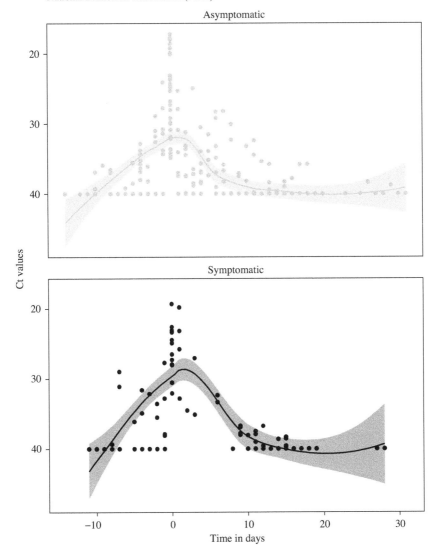

Figure 3.2. Viral load within NBA players, including those infected asymptomatically (upper panel) and symptomatically (lower panel) as a function of time in days. *Source*: Data from Kissler, S.M., et al. (2021). Viral dynamics of acute SARS-CoV-2 infection and applications to diagnostic and public health strategies. *PLOS Biology* 19: e3001333. https://doi.org/10.1371/journal.pbio.3001333. Visualization from Park, S.W., et al. (2022). Intermediate levels of asymptomatic transmission can lead to the highest levels of epidemic fatalities. MedRxiv. https://doi.org/10.1101/2022.08.01 .22278288. Licensed under Creative Commons BY 4.0 DEED, Attribution 4.0 International. https://creativecommons.org/licenses/by/4.0/.

This figure shows the "Ct" levels from PCR-based viral tests as a function of the days since peak viral load of NBA players. The data was collected as part of a preventative strategy in which the NBA set up a "bubble" to limit the introduction of COVID-19 into staff and player communities and to rapidly identify infections before they had a chance to catalyze new clusters.[12] As already explained, it is both possible and common that someone can feel fine and have a positive result on a PCR test—this is especially relevant for otherwise healthy young adults (as described in chapter 2). If the viral load in the sample is already high, then it takes fewer doubling cycles to reach a critical level to be detected in a PCR-based molecular viral test. This is what the Ct level represents: it is the "cycle threshold" for detection. Fewer cycles means more virus was present in the sample, and more cycles means less virus was present in the sample. As should be apparent, individuals who are asymptomatically infected can sometimes have higher viral loads than those who are symptomatically infected. Moreover, a proxy for the duration of infectiousness—measured as the time above a critical Ct value—can be nearly as long for asymptomatic individuals as for symptomatic individuals. But viral load is only part of the story. Behavior matters, too.

In the spring and summer of 2020, many people began new daily walking routines to undo the monotony of at-home work, online schools, and social isolation. A cough or a sneeze was, then at least, considered a potential sign of being infected. This kind of self-diagnosis of symptoms has a practical effect. Individuals with symptoms are likely to reduce their interactions with others as a direct function of their symptomatic state. But, if infectiousness is uncorrelated to infectious state (or at least decoupled), then asymptomatic infections can be just as important in driving COVID-19 spread, making it difficult, if not nearly impossible, to stop.

Individuals who feel fine are unlikely to need a day off. They go out to work, visit friends and family, and are more likely to let their guard down when around others. Why should someone who feels fine need to wear a mask when around others? That is, of course, a rhetorical question, but it is a question that must be asked—and answered. If we knew that someone who felt fine was not infectious, then they would not pose a risk to others if they took off a mask in indoor settings. Of course, they would then have a far higher chance of getting infected if others were shedding viruses. In contrast, someone with symptoms is far more likely to stay home.

To move from one particular infection to many requires a different way of thinking. It requires taking a population-scale approach—the approach we will explore next.

From Individuals to Populations—the Ascent

The transmissibility of any disease depends on many factors, including which fraction of the population is vulnerable to infection. In the case of SARS-CoV-2, the answer is that all of us were almost certainly immunologically naive at the beginning of the outbreak. Our immune systems had not seen the shapes of viral envelopes that can be recognized as antigens and then specifically eliminated by our immune system. This early assumption of population-scale vulnerability was correct, despite speculation that widespread asymptomatic infections might be a direct consequence of cross-immunity from coronaviruses that cause the common cold.[13] As a result, when a handful or perhaps hundreds, if not thousands, of SARS-CoV-2 virus particles entered into someone's nasal passageways and lungs, those viruses were not immediately recognized as "foreign" by the immune system. Instead, these newly introduced viruses were more likely to encounter and bind to target cells inside the lugs. At this point, the virus would begin to take over the cell, replicate, make more virus particles, and then spread from one target cell to many, causing an active infection that could then trigger the released of infectious SARS-CoV-2 particles through the air.[14]

We can quantify the extent to which one individual infects others in terms of both the time and number of new individuals infected. Consider the introduction of COVID-19 into an otherwise susceptible community. In late December 2019 and January 2020, this would have corresponded to the first cases of COVID-19 in Wuhan.[15] In January and February 2020, the same type of process unfolded in Italy, with an epicenter in the Lombardy region (as described earlier in chapter 1). In February and March 2020, the very same process unfolded in Seattle, New York, Los Angeles, and soon throughout the United States.[16,17] In each region, an initial individual was infected and then infected a few others. Dating the start and source of infections in a particular focal region is an area of ongoing research.[18] Nonetheless, if one infected person traveling to a focal region were to infect three others, and then those three infect three more, and so on, within a few weeks and certainly months the outbreak would reach hundreds, thousands, and beyond.

Transmission of a virus requires both means and opportunity. The means corresponds to whether or not an individual is infectious—actively shedding virus particles—irrespective of symptoms. The opportunity is determined by whether or not an infectious person is close enough to a susceptible person to transmit the disease. In the case of a respiratory pathogen like SARS-CoV-2, the transmission route is predominantly through the air (as explored in detail in chapter 2). Being "close" need not mean being in the same room at the same time. An infectious individual can release virus particles into the air that linger so that a susceptible individual can become infected even if they are alone. For example, in one notable case of suspected airborne transmission, a traveler managed to infect multiple individuals staying across the hall in a quarantine hotel in New Zealand; surveillance footage revealed that their only known "contact" was when the infectious individual and the susceptible individual opened their quarantine hotel room doors at nearly the same time.[19]

We can use these elements—means and opportunity—to scale up what happens at individual levels to the larger population. The purpose in doing so is to estimate how many individuals might become infected in the population based on transmission between individuals. If we know that and something about the chances that an infected case becomes severe, then we are a step closer to understanding the overall threat of a particular emerging infectious disease—including Ebola virus disease, SARS-1, and yes, SARS-CoV-2.

Keeping track of epidemiological models will require that we name a few concepts. We will call the period in which an individual can infect others the *average duration of infectiousness*. Duration varies by individuals. For some individuals, this period will last 7 days, whereas for others it may be 4 days or 14 days. We will call the average number of new infections caused by a single infectious individual in an otherwise susceptible population the *basic reproduction number*. Likewise, despite using the average value for the sake of models, it is important to recognize that the actual number of secondary cases caused by a primary case will vary. For some, it will be three, whereas for others it will be one, five, or even none at all. These two numbers—the duration of infectiousness and the basic reproduction number—are essential in determining how fast a disease will spread and how severe an outbreak will become. To reiterate: we should not expect that these two numbers are the same for every person in a population (nor are they the only two numbers relevant in scaling up epidemic estimates). Some people may only shed virus for a few days; others (in rare cases) may shed virus for a few weeks. Likewise, some infectious individuals may infect no one at all, whereas some infectious individuals may infect many more, even dozens, as has been documented in superspreading events in the United States and elsewhere.[20]

For now, then, we should think of the duration of infectiousness and the basic reproduction number as appropriate averages. The advantage of this kind of simplification is that it allows us to make the connection between the individual and the population, even if we must use caution, acknowledging that such estimates will be guides that must be refined later on.

Let us start with a single infectious individual who infects 3 other individuals (on average) over the course of approximately one week. In the second week, those 3 individuals infect a total of 9 people before they are no longer infectious. In the third week, those 9 individuals infect a total of 27 people before they are no longer infectious. And so on. In reality, the timing of the infections are not demarcated into different "generations" (i.e., the primary, secondary, tertiary, and so on). Instead, the generations of infections overlap so that the focal individual could infect person A on day 1, and then person A could infect someone else before the focal individual infects person B.

The key here is that an individual infects more than one person, on average. This means that even as the individual recovers (or, in the rare case, dies), there is still more than one newly infectious person in the population. As long as each individual causes at least one new infection on average, the disease can grow and grow and grow. The particular choice of the number 3 in this example depends on the disease (it is lower for Ebola, about right for COVID-19, and higher for measles).[21] More generally, this number holds a special place in epidemic theory as the basic reproduction number (i.e., the average number of new infections caused by a single infectious individual, on average, in an otherwise susceptible population). Here, we will refer to it as R_0 (see the glossary for more information on the reproduction number and other technical terms).[22,23,24] As long as R_0 exceeds 1, then the disease is expected to spread.

This rapid—indeed exponential—increase will continue to unfold until something happens. In classical epidemiological studies, the "something" that happens is that the virus runs out of individuals to infect.

If one individual infects three people, on average, as do those three people, and so on, then the number of susceptible individuals who are vulnerable to infection declines as individuals recover, first by one, then by three, then by nine, and so on. If we assume the individuals who recover from infection are immune to reinfection (at least on the timescales of the epidemic wave), then the effective number of new infections will progressively decrease. In other words, the assumption that everyone is vulnerable to infection becomes less appropriate the more people who are infected. The same holds true for forest fires, insofar that a fire burning in a dense forest can burn up the very fuel needed for its spread.[25] Figure 3.3 illustrates the point.

These three sketches illustrate the progressive change in disease status of individuals in a population—whether susceptible (S), infectious (I), or recovered and presumably immune (R). At each point, figure 3.3 highlights the interactions between a focal infectious individual given variation in the fraction P of the population that has already been infected. At the start, P is 0—the population is immunologically naive.

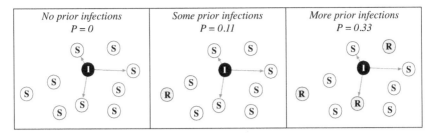

Figure 3.3. Illustration of depletion of susceptibles during an outbreak. In this example, an infectious individual (I) interacts with a population that includes both susceptible (S) and recovered and presumably immune (R) individuals. At the start, the fraction of individuals that are recovered is 0, and then over time, as individuals are infected and recover, this number increases to 0.11 (approximately 1 in 9) and then to 0.33 (approximately 1 in 3).

Now, consider an individual who is infected much farther along in the outbreak such that P is now greater than 0. If this focal individual were to interact with 300 individuals in a week, and there was a 1 in 100 chance that a contact could lead to an infection, there would be less than 3 individuals infected on average. Why? Because there is only a (1–P) probability that these 3 individuals had not yet been infected. If P was 0.33 (or 1 in 3), as in the last panel in the figure, this means that 1 in 3 individuals had already been infected. In that case, the onward transmission from a focal individual would lead to 2 new infections instead of 3. The disease outbreak would still increase in size, but more slowly. But, at some point, if the fraction of previously infected individuals P becomes high enough, then the onward transmission from a focal individual would lead to just 1 new infection, on average.

This presents a critical threshold limit—in theory. It is the point where infections operate at a replacement level. Rather than increasing in numbers, the disease should begin to plateau and then descend and disappear altogether.

From Individuals to Populations—the Descent

The spread of a disease can lead to exponential growth as one individual spreads to a few contacts, and then those newly infected contacts spread to even more. Yet, such exponential growth cannot go on forever. First, contacts are structured. Each of us is more likely to interact and share the same air with individuals in our household and in our places of work than with someone living in a distant state or city.[26] Second, outside of family or social networks, there are many people who we will nonetheless interact with in transit, in stores, in offices, and other indoor locations. The potential for COVID-19's initial spread was based on early estimates that each of us could potentially infect three other individuals, on average.[27] In reality, there was significant variation in this number, reflecting mobility patterns, individual choices (e.g., whether a person wore a mask or not), and the duration of infectiousness. Even give some variation, epidemic models share a common feature: they predict that at some point, enough individuals will have been infected that a newly infectious individual is unlikely to amplify the size of the ongoing outbreak.

The decline of epidemics occurs through a process called "susceptible depletion," the incipient steps of which are described in the previous section. Over time, the average number of new infections caused by a single infectious individual should decrease because there are fewer susceptible people for any newly infectious person to infect. But, how much lower should the "effective" reproduction number go? As figure 3.3 explains, as more of the population is infected and recovers, then a smaller fraction, $1-P$, remains susceptible. This means that the effective reproduction number (or R_{eff}) is equal to the product of the basic reproduction number R_0 and the susceptible fraction $(1-P)$. If R_0 is 3 and $P = 2/3$, then the product of $3 \times (1-2/3)$ is equal to 1. At this point, one infectious individual no longer generates at least one infectious individual on average such that cases begin to stall and then decrease. This is termed *herd immunity*. Figure 3.4 illustrates this point for the case $P = 2/3$ and $R_0 = 3$.

The herd immunity threshold is the level of prior infections such that a single new case leads to just one new case on average. The value of herd immunity varies depending on the pathogen and the context

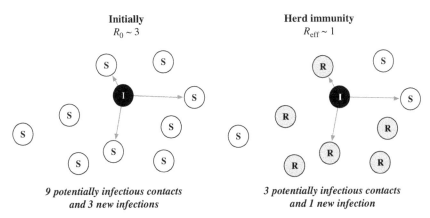

Initially
$R_0 \sim 3$

Herd immunity
$R_{\text{eff}} \sim 1$

9 potentially infectious contacts
and 3 new infections

3 potentially infectious contacts
and 1 new infection

Figure 3.4. Illustration of how susceptible depletion can lead to a decrease in incidence over time. The left side considers one infectious individual (black circle marked with the letter I) who infects three new individuals (circles connected by arrows). The right side shows the same circumstance, only now two of the three individuals who would otherwise have been newly infected are no longer susceptible to infection (recovered individuals are marked with the letter R). As a result, only one individual becomes newly infected.

(and, ultimately, behavior); it denotes a fraction of individuals who must be infected before susceptibles are depleted so that one case does not lead to more than one case, on average. After that point, the incidence declines. Incidence denotes the number of new cases per unit time. The reason is that once the product of $R_0 \times (1-P)$ drops below one, then there will be more circumstances where a single infectious individual does not infect anyone at all. For example, if the effective reproduction number is 0.95, then 95 of 100 infectious individuals may infect 1 more person, whereas 5 of those 100 infectious individuals will infect no one at all. As a result, the number of infectious individuals (and the associated incidence) begins to decline.

We can put all of these ideas together by developing a simplified representation of epidemic dynamics that occur at population scales. To do so, we can think of the population in aggregate in terms of the *fractions* of individuals that are susceptible, exposed, infectious, or recovered. Whereas individual outcomes may differ, the characteristic spread of a disease in a well-connected population predicts three distinct phases.

- The first "growth" phase: infectious spread in a largely naive population leads to exponential growth in infectious individuals and, soon thereafter, in recovered individuals. Even though the number of infectious individuals is growing rapidly, the absolute numbers of currently or previously infected are relatively small compared to the total population.
- The second "plateau" phase: the cumulative number of infected individuals (whether currently or previously) grows so large that the infectious curve begins to flatten—similar to what William Farr noticed in reports of smallpox deaths in nineteenth-century England, as discussed in Chapter 1. As a result, the number of infectious individuals reach a peak—this corresponds to the population having reached a herd immunity threshold.
- The third "decline" phase: after the population has crossed a herd immunity threshold, then the infection starts to decay nearly as quickly as it increased. Notably, not everyone is infected. Epidemic models predict that there will still be a subpopulation of individuals who are never infected, for reasons of circumstance, i.e., they were not infected initially and by the end, they are protected by population immunity.[28]

These three phases can be seen in figure 3.5, which represents a synthetic simulation of disease dynamics using only two rules: (i) infectious and susceptible individuals come into contact at random, leading sometimes to a new infection; (ii) infectious individuals ultimately recover. This is referred to as an SIR model after its three "compartments" (Susceptible, Infectious, and Recovered/Removed). These models can be extended into SEIR models depending on whether an exposed (E) compartment is included—referring to the incubation phase. In this example, approximately 94% of the population is infected by the end of the epidemic.

The herd immunity threshold is a population-scale feature that depends on individual transmission features. The herd immunity

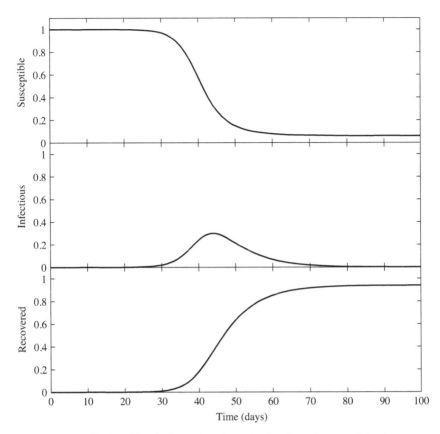

Figure 3.5. Synthetic epidemic dynamics where the fraction of susceptibles decreases (top) as the fraction of infectious individuals increases (middle) and the fraction of recovered individuals (bottom) also increases and eventually plateaus. Simulation includes $R_0 = 3$ and an infectious period of 6 days. The disease has a peak approximately 42 days after the initial outbreak.

threshold is also the first estimate of the potential size of an outbreak—and sets the stage for assessing the total severity of an outbreak once we include asymptomatic spread. As a result of exponential spread, what may seem like a small number of new transmissions per individual (e.g., an R_0 value of 3) can generate a tidal wave of cases infecting far more than two-thirds of the population. The actual size will be even larger than the herd immunity threshold because of epidemic overshoot (figure 3.6).

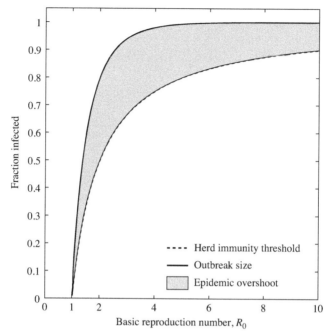

Figure 3.6. Outbreak size measured in terms of the fraction of the population infected as a function of the basic reproduction number, R_0. The solid line denotes the final outbreak size as a fraction of the population. The dashed line denotes the herd immunity threshold (HIT), where one individual is likely to cause only one new infection on average. When R_0 is 2, then the HIT level is 0.5; when R_0 is 3, then the HIT level is 0.67; when R_0 is 4, then the HIT level is 0.75, and so on. Once susceptibles have been depleted to the HIT, the incidence of new cases is expected to decrease. The final size is always above the HIT size and approaches (but does not reach) 1 as the basic reproduction number increases. A basic reproduction number of 1 denotes a threshold—below which an outbreak is not expected to occur. The difference between the curves is the epidemic overshoot.

Epidemic overshoot is the phenomena whereby cumulative cases increase substantially even after the population reaches the herd immunity threshold. To see why, imagine a population in which 66% have been infected, given a disease whose basic reproduction number is 3. Once this level of the population is infected, then any newly infected individual will cause one (or fewer) new cases, on average. But these new cases still accumulate and can cause harm. As a result, the cumulative cases will go up even higher—well beyond 66%—until finally the disease fades away and the outbreak stops. In the example of figure 3.6, the expected final size of the epidemic exceeds 90% when R_0 is 3 (this basic reproduction number is close to initial estimates for SARS-CoV-2),[29] and it goes up with increasing R_0.

Striving, reaching, or pushing for herd immunity has at times appeared to be a strategy proposed by political leaders in the United States,[30] the United Kingdom,[31] and Sweden.[32] The rationale is that if enough healthy individuals acquire immunity, then those most at risk will be protected. Such strategies have, at times, been supported by medical doctors,[33] economists,[34] and even Nobel Prize winners[35] as the basis for predicting the imminent end to the pandemic—only to be proved wrong.[36] Such advocacy minimized the life-and-death consequences of achieving herd immunity through infections and not from vaccination. Perhaps its advocates were simply confused, or perhaps they were just cynical. Either way, they were wrong.

What is in fact good about population immunity? Population immunity tracks the level of susceptible depletion in a population. As population immunity increases, then the fraction of individuals who are vulnerable to infection decreases. Higher levels of population immunity mean that a smaller fraction of individuals can get infected (and sick) when exposed. There are two principal mechanisms to acquire individual immunity and, in turn, to accumulate population immunity. The first is through infections. The second is through vaccinations. The failure of striving for herd immunity as a public health response policy stems from simple arithmetic, mixed with some understanding of population-scale outcomes.

Given that the R_0 of COVID-19 was estimated to be approximately 3, then unmitigated spread could lead to upwards of 90% of the population infected (in theory). This number comes with caveats, given that the total size of an outbreak depends on multiple assumptions about how people interact, who they interact with, and whether or not they can become reinfected, and can often differ substantially from simple epidemic predictions.[37] Nonetheless, the magnitude of spread provides a baseline for moving from individual-level transmission to population-level severity.[38] Caveats notwithstanding, the R_0 of 3 for COVID-19 implied that perhaps 300 million Americans would be infected. Of these, if 1 in 100 individuals die, the implication is that the United States could experience 3 million deaths. What happens if both of these estimates were twofold too severe? In that case, there might still be 750,000 total fatalities. In reality, there were more than 1 million documented fatalities in the United States alone due to COVID-19 in a little more than two years since the outbreak began. Hence, in the United States, the cumulative effect of silent transmission and public policy failures led to outcomes that were broadly anticipated in early 2020.[39] These scenarios were presented as a caution to take action and give more time to reach herd immunity the safe and ethical way: through vaccinations.

Indeed, these estimates point out why herd immunity can be good, if obtained through population-scale vaccination campaigns. For a disease with a basic reproduction number of 3, then the herd immunity level is 2/3. That is, ~66% of the population should have immunity such that one case does not lead to more than one case, on average. This, then, is the benefit of vaccination. If more than two-thirds of the population could be effectively vaccinated (a topic examined in greater detail in part 2 of this book), then in theory, there would be no meaningful outbreaks—and no large-scale fatalities. The word "effectively" is doing a lot of work here. It implies a vaccination campaign that reaches the breadth and diversity of the population in all senses. But it highlights a key point. One need not vaccinate everyone to provide individual protection to those who have been vaccinated and population immunity even to those who are not vaccinated (or those who are vaccinated but do not mount sufficiently robust immune responses to be protected). Measles, polio, and pertussis (whooping cough) are clarion examples of how universal childhood vaccinations can dramatically halt otherwise devasting diseases in their tracks.

Yet, in early 2020, vaccines against SARS-CoV-2 were not yet available. The fact that effective vaccines became available less than a year later is truly remarkable.[40] The failure of governments and the public to adequately vaccinate populations is also truly remarkable, but not in the same sense.[41] Instead, the pandemic raged, abetted in part by a misleading hope that herd immunity could help. In the absence of a vaccine, paths toward herd immunity come only with many infections, many severe cases, and far too many fatalities. The spread of COVID-19 was made more complicated by a seemingly incongruous fact: many people seemed to have exceptionally mild or even asymptomatic courses of infection. These asymptomatic infections were SARS-CoV-2's secret weapon. We must now unpack precisely why asymptomatic *transmission* can in fact worsen population-level outcomes.

Disease Severity at the Population Scale

Scientist do not yet fully understand what determines the fate of a viral infection. Why do two people, of similar age and health levels, have widely disparate outcomes? Why do children and young adults have predominantly mild courses of infection while the likelihood of severity increases rapidly with age? Even if there is a statistical tendency, why do two people with apparently similar profiles—similar ages, health, and comorbidities—have totally different outcomes? What are the chance events that set these outcomes? Is the outcome determined by the initial viral dose, genetic factors, the status of the individual's immune system—or perhaps some combination of all of these factors? Yet one thing is certain, irrespective of the severity of the outcome: transmission can occur irrespective of symptoms.

In order to connect individual- and population-level outcomes, we have to extend the framework introduced in the previous section while accommodating alternative modes of infection: both asymptomatic and symptomatic. Doing so will help to reveal the epidemiological mechanism by which intermediate levels of asymptomatic transmission act to worsen the severity of the outbreak at population scales.

But first, we have to set a ground rule. This ground rule will become a guide throughout this book, both in terms of explaining why we failed to stop COVID-19 and why we must establish priorities for what public health interventions are trying to do in the first place.

Severity matters.

The severity of an outbreak at the population scale should be measured by the aggregate number of severe outcomes at the individual level. Perhaps there should be more ground rules, but the success or failure of policy interventions should depend on keeping track of this rule.

There are many metrics of severity. Individuals who are hospitalized with a COVID-19 infection and, in particular, those who are intubated often face long-term and chronic post-recovery challenges. Sustained loss of lung function or neurophysiological damage represents the kind of severe outcome that public health interventions must try and prevent. Likewise, an individual who recovers from a "mild" infection but later experiences debilitating and sustained physical damage that had gone unnoticed—whether neurophysiological or physical—represents another example of a severe outcome. "Long COVID" remains a key topic for ongoing research and interventions.[42] But, for now, we will focus on aggregate fatalities as a barometer of disease severity as a means to connect asymptomatic transmission with the overall severity of the COVID-19 outbreak—especially in the early stages of the pandemic.

In order to assess the prevaccination fatality risk, it is worth revisiting the cumulative numbers of cases and fatalities in 2020 alone. Consider two early examples, one from Georgia and one from New York City. There were about 11,000 documented fatalities with ~650,000 reported infections as of January 1, 2021, in Georgia.[43] In New York City, there were approximately 25,000 documented fatalities out of 450,000 documented cases as of January 1, 2021.[44] Dividing the number of documented fatalities by the number of documented cases yields a case fatality rate (CFR) of 1.6% in Georgia and 5.6% in New York City. But significant caution is warranted before interpreting these fatality percentages as the risk of dying if you are infected. CFR is a meaningful number as long as cases are well-ascertained. In practice, both the numerator (the deaths) and the denominator (the cases) in the CFR estimate can be incorrect. For COVID-19, the number of cases was a significant underestimate of the true number of infections (deaths were also underestimated but not to the same extent). As a result, if one is interested in estimating the risk of dying from an infection, then the CFR divides deaths by too small a number (dividing by documented cases, rather than actual infections). As a result, estimates using raw deaths divided by raw cases represent significant overestimates of the ratio of disease-induced fatalities by total infections (i.e., the infection fatality rate, or IFR). For COVID-19, the IFR was far smaller than the CFR.[45] It is an issue that was magnified in intense outbreaks at the start of the pandemic (like in New York City).

Figuring out if one had or has a SARS-CoV-2 infection has not been easy. In most of the world, it is simply impossible to identify the majority of infections because of the lack of access to timely and accurate testing. The same holds for the United States. The levels of testing have varied both over time and between regions, yet these differences must be resolved in any effort to prepare and prevent the next pandemic. As just one example, on April 11, 2020, there were 730 total fatalities attributed to COVID-19 in New York City (including documented deaths and deaths in which COVID-19 was the probable cause). Let us envision, for a moment, that the case fatality rate was largely unchanged throughout 2020—in the United States, there were ~335,000 COVID-19 documented fatalities and 20,000,000 cases.[46] This ratio is approximately ~1.6%. If this CFR was in fact the same as the IFR, then there should be a 1 in 60 chance of dying from infection. That would mean that it would require ~44,000 new infections every day near the end of March so that two to three weeks later—accounting for the incubation period of the infection, the development of symptoms, hospitalization, and (sometimes) treatment in an intensive care unit—730 of those people would die of COVID-19. Yet, on a typical day in late March 2020, there were only 2,000 to 5,000 individuals who were documented as being infected with COVID-19 in New York City. This does not mean that COVID-19 was somehow more lethal. Instead, it means that the denominator was way off, by a factor that is at least 10-fold, if not even higher.

Over time, testing did improve, and it even transformed in practice from expensive lab-based PCR tests to relatively inexpensive at-home antigen tests. But improvement was not enough. For the bulk of the pandemic, testing capacity was inadequate. There were not enough tests for all who wanted to take one. Critically, access to tests could take time—significant time. In one example, passengers had to wait for hours in their cars to access drive-through testing centers in Texas.[47] Not everyone can access such testing centers. Even if they can, fewer yet can afford to lose hours in a day waiting to get tested. And, even if folks manage to get tested, the backlog in lab capacity meant that multiday waits to get results were typical. The aggregate impact of such capacity failures meant that testing was largely used to confirm symptomatic cases—that is, as a molecular diagnostic. Over time, the CDC (and other groups) estimated there were 4 actual cases for every 1 documented case.[48] That would imply that if the CFR was 1.6%, then the actual fatality rate should be fourfold lower.

In summary, although raw CFR estimates would suggest that COVID-19 has a 1% to 6% chance of causing a fatality, improvements in accounting for mild and asymptomatic infections, which are far less likely to be documented, suggest that the IFR is closer to 0.5%, or 1 in 200 individuals across the age distribution of the US population. So, to estimate the severity of SARS-CoV-2 at the population level requires one more piece of the puzzle: the total number of individuals infected.

In this chapter, we introduced the core mechanisms by which disease transmission between individuals can lead to a large-scale outbreak at the population level. The central idea is that transmission between susceptible and infectious individuals can lead to a rapid, exponential increase in infections that then plateaus and eventually diminishes over time. In the case of COVID-19, however, the rapid spread also brought large numbers of fatalities and behavior change—including changes in mobility and how people behaved in public settings. Therefore, a plateau does not necessarily mean that there are no more susceptible individuals; it may mean that in a largely vulnerable population, people are changing their behavior, e.g., by social distancing and wearing masks.

Behavior change was also influenced by COVID-19 related mandates. Lockdowns were imposed state by state between March and April 2020. In this period, individuals were expected to stay at home unless they were considered frontline or essential workers. Mobility reports using data collected from mobile phones indicated a 50% (or more) decrease in travel frequency to businesses and retail stores during the spring and summer 2020.[49] Yet, going out to the grocery store or a pharmacy was unavoidable for many people, and rapidly, the definition of who was an essential worker began to expand. In response, individuals began to use masks, both in advance of and because of mask mandates imposed by state authorities. The net effect was apparent. In February 2020, very few people wore a mask in public. By late March 2020, mask-wearing became more commonplace. The first statewide mask mandates were imposed in early April 2020 (e.g., in New Jersey).[50] A number of similar orders followed, largely in solidly Democratic or Democratic-leaning states (figure 3.7). By early summer 2020, the majority of Americans reported using a mask most or all of the time when in a store or business.[51] In total, 39 of 50 states would issue a combination of executive and court orders requiring that masks be worn in stores and businesses, although enforceability, interpretation, and duration of orders varied significantly between states and over time.[52] A CDC-commissioned survey showed rapid increases in mask use between early April and mid-May.[53] Notably, individuals older than 65 years reported using a mask only 37% of the time when in public settings in the week leading up to the April 2020 survey. In contrast, that percentage had increased to 79% by mid-May.

This data illustrates a central point missing in curve-fits to epidemic death data, such as the Institute for Health Metrics and Evaluation (IHME) model (discussed in chapter 1), and in mechanistic models of unmitigated spread (as introduced earlier in this chapter): people can change their behavior in response to a disease threat. There are many ways to include such reactions, but here, we will add perhaps the most readily apparent ingredient to the mix of relevance to COVID-19. We will assume that a fraction of individuals who are symptomatic will take precautions and that asymptomatically infected individuals will not take such precautions because they are unaware they are infected.

To explore this scenario, let us take an extreme assumption—that 100% of symptomatic individuals become aware of symptoms, that transmission depends on symptoms, and so symptomatic individuals isolate with the onset of symptoms and do not infect others. It is an idealized world, but the benefits of exploring such idealized scenarios

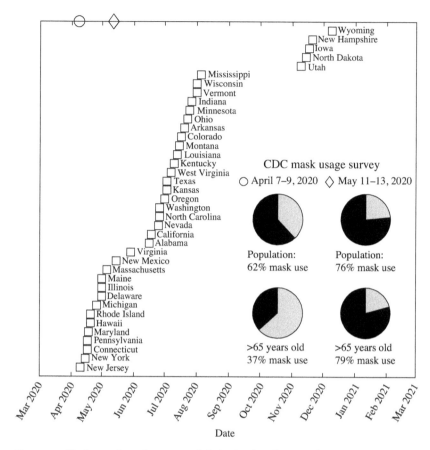

Figure 3.7. Mask mandates by state and their timeline for introduction, according to statewide executive orders and/or court orders for mask use in public settings. The four pie charts show the results of a mask usage survey conducted by the CDC, during April 7–9, 2020, and May 11–13, 2020, denoting the fraction of individuals in the general population (top) and those >65 years of age (bottom) that reported using a mask in public in the week before the survey. Black = mask used; gray = mask unused. *Sources:* Ballotpedia. (2022). State-level mask requirements in response to the coronavirus (COVID-19) pandemic, 2020–2022. https://ballotpedia.org/State -level_mask_requirements_in_response_to_the_coronavirus_(COVID-19) _pandemic,_2020-2022. Mask usage survey data is from Fisher, K.A., et al. (2020). Factors associated with cloth face covering use among adults during the COVID-19 pandemic—United States, April and May 2020. *MMWR* 69: 933–937. https://doi.org /10.15585/mmwr.mm6928e3.

is that they can shed light on outcomes even in realistic cases. Likewise, we will assume that asymptomatic individuals will carry on as normal—unaware of their infection state.

Let us start again with a single infectious individual in an otherwise susceptible population. For convenience, we will say that the person has an asymptomatic infection. In this particular example, we will assume that in the absence of behavior change, the basic reproduction number is 4 (a higher number than used before that allows for simpler calculations). As a result, the focal infectious individual is unaware of their disease status and infects four other people. Of those four, two have symptomatic infections, and one has an asymptomatic infection. Because symptomatically infected individuals isolate upon symptom onset, those two symptomatically infected individuals do not infect anyone else. But the two individuals who have asymptomatic infections do interact normally and infect four more people each, or eight in total, of which four are asymptomatically infected and four are symptomatically infected. This process continues. Table 3.1 presents the idealized spread and characteristics over multiple disease "generations."

Table 3.1. Epidemic dynamics in an idealized spread over multiple generations

Generation	Asymptomatic	Symptomatic	Fatalities (average)
0	1	0	0
1	2	2	0.02
2	4	4	0.04
3	8	8	0.08
4	16	16	0.16
5	32	32	0.32
6	64	64	0.64
7	128	128	1.28
8	256	256	2.56
Total	511	510	5

Note: Each asymptomatic individual causes four new infections, of which 50% are asymptomatic, assuming that symptomatic individuals do not cause new infections. The last row denotes the cumulative number of asymptomatic infections, symptomatic cases, and fatalities. (Because of the low case fatality rate, the last row lists the approximate number of fatalities.) The arrows denote the transmission events from asymptomatic individuals and the chance that symptomatic infections lead to fatalities.

The table's arrows illustrate the potential gap between what is driving new infections (the asymptomatic) and what is driving new fatalities (the symptomatic).

Beyond generation 1, the number of cases increases by a factor of 2, despite the fact that R_0 is 4. This is because only half of those infected can infect others. Hence, there are 4 infections at generation 1, 8 in generation 2, 16 in generation 3, and so on. Of these, half are symptomatic, and 1% of symptomatic cases die. This means that over eight disease generations, a single infectious individual could generate a transmission chain that leads to more than 1,000 cumulative infections of which ~500 were symptomatic and ~5 were fatal (a 1% CFR). If the disease generations take about one week, on average, then in two months, an emerging infectious disease could start to become visible in terms of population-level impacts. This process holds for the next eight generations, so that two months after that, there might be more than 100,000 active cases and more than 1,000 total fatalities. Exponentials are fast. Yet this illustration raises a question and another extreme limit. What happens when 100% of the infections are asymptomatic?

Table 3.2 reveals a completely different story. When all infections are asymptomatic, the disease now spreads faster, leading to more than 2,000 infections over 8 generations. But, because all the infections are asymptomatic, by definition there are no fatalities. It should be apparent that if our objective is to take preventative steps to minimize

Table 3.2. Epidemic dynamics when 100% of infections are asymptomatic and each infectious individuals infects four others, on average

Generation	Asymptomatic	Symptomatic	Fatalities (average)
0	1	0	0
1	4	0	0
2	16	0	0
3	32	0	0
4	64	0	0
5	128	0	0
6	256	0	0
7	512	0	0
8	1,024	0	0
Total	2,047	0	0

fatalities, then no further action is needed. Although this model is oversimplified, we are already familiar with diseases that exclusively cause mild or asymptomatic infections (e.g., the common cold). Many of the causative agents of the common cold are coronaviruses—the same family of viruses that causes both SARS-1[54] and SARS-CoV-2.[55] Seasonal coronaviruses cause mild infections with symptoms including runny nose, aches, and cough that may induce someone to stay home from school, work, or social events. The common cold does not and should not induce public lockdowns.

There is one more part of the puzzle required. Let us now assume that asymptomatic infections are absent. Instead, all individuals who are infected are symptomatic, and transmission can be stopped if symptomatic individuals isolate. Using the same approach as before, in the event that someone is incidentally infected, there is little to no possibility for the disease to spread. The table is simpler (see table 3.3). A symptomatic individual may die rarely, but they will not infect others. Hence, at the population scale, the disease has little impact.

These three examples can be encapsulated as follows. When all infections are asymptomatic, then the individual and population outcomes coincide: the disease is not severe, causing no harm to the population when we measure harm in terms of total fatalities. When all infections are symptomatic, then the disease may cause significant harm to the infected person and even end in a fatal outcome, but it is unlikely to spread to others. It is the intermediate case—where some individuals have asymptomatic outcomes and others have symptomatic outcomes—that leads to the worst outcomes for the population as a whole.

Table 3.3. Epidemic dynamics when 100% of infections are symptomatic and infected individuals do not transmit it to others because of behavior change tied to symptom onset

Generation	Asymptomatic	Symptomatic	Fatalities (average)
0	0	1	0.01
1	0	0	0
Total	0	1	~0

Why Asymptomatic Transmission Leads to Increased Fatalities

The previous examples contain the kernel of a bona fide epidemiological paradox. But they are also extreme in their assumptions. More generally, it is possible to formalize the link between asymptomatic transmission at individual scales and pandemic severity at population scales using an outbreak model that incorporates all of these elements in one place (figure 3.8).

These ingredients are built on standard assumptions in mathematical models of an epidemic; they are used to simulate how an epidemic might spread. Figure 3.9 shows what happens when all of these ingredients come together in a simulation of an epidemic with different levels of reduction in disease transmission from symptomatic individuals relative to asymptomatic individuals.[56] The x-axis of in each panel denotes changes in the fraction of individuals who are asymptomatic—denoted by the variable p. The asymptomatic fraction ranges from 0 (all are symptomatic) to 1 (all are asymptomatic). The y-axis in each panel denotes the total number of fatalities in a population with

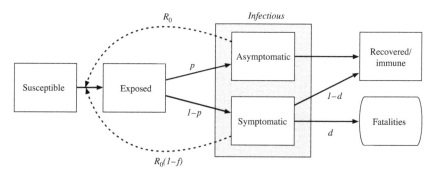

Figure 3.8. Example rules of epidemic modeling and asymptomatic transmission. The baseline transmissibility of the disease is R_0 (i.e., infectious individuals can infect R_0 other individuals, on average, in an otherwise susceptible population). Newly infected individuals have a probability p of having an asymptomatic infection and a probability $1-p$ of having a symptomatic infection. Symptomatically infected individuals reduce their risk of transmission (e.g., through mask-wearing or isolation) by a factor $(1-f)$ relative to asymptomatic individuals. Symptomatically infected individuals die a fraction d of the time (e.g., 1 in 100).

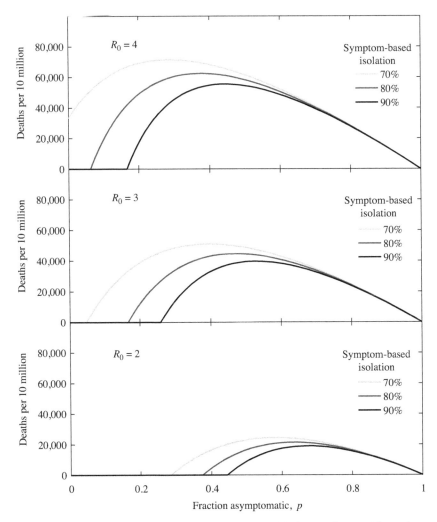

Figure 3.9. Estimated fatalities in a mathematical model of an epidemic with varying fractions of individual cases that are asymptomatic (x-axis). The fatalities per 10 million are presented on the y-axis. The panels consider R_0 values of 2 (bottom), 3 (middle), and 4 (top), with varying levels of symptom-based isolation. In all cases, the peak fatalities occur for intermediate values of p.

10 million individuals (somewhat larger than New York City and slightly smaller than Georgia).

The takeaway is straightforward: *Fatalities peak at intermediate levels of the fraction of asymptomatic infection.*

This result reflects the tension between outcomes at the individual and population levels. The simulations represent a sequence of steps that are included, with variation, at the core of modern, epidemiological simulation initiatives.[57] The inclusion of asymptomatic transmission has also been the source of a practical problem that explains why COVID-19 has been such a formidable pathogen. A respiratory illness that infects individuals causing mild (or no) symptoms yet transmits to others is difficult to stop. Asymptomatic individuals become hubs of infection while symptomatic individuals are the visible nodes in such infection chains. Asymptomatic and symptomatic individuals may have nearly the same potential for transmission but very different behavioral responses. This difference implies that intermediate levels of asymptomatic infections tend to fuel accelerated spread. Even worse, if asymptomatic or mild infections are sufficiently common, then it can lead to a perception gap.

In this particular set of examples, the peak fatality rate happens when approximately 30% to 70% of individuals have asymptomatic infections. This is precisely the relevant range for SARS-CoV-2. Yet, even this result understates how much the asymptomatic route of infections makes the disease worse in aggregate.

Individuals who are infected go through different stages of an infection. After exposure and infection, the virus begins to replicate but remains at sufficiently low levels that the individual is not considered infectious. Instead, such individuals are considered "exposed." The term "exposed" simply denotes the staged progression of the disease. The next stage can be asymptomatic or symptomatic. In either case, such individuals are infectious. Some individuals who are asymptomatic will remain so and then recover without exhibiting signs consistent with standard thresholds for symptoms. But other individuals will shift from an asymptomatic stage to a symptomatic stage. So, while accounting for the spread of COVID-19 the role of asymptomatic transmission shapes outcomes in two key ways. First, some individuals never get symptoms and nonetheless transmit. Second, some individuals start off asymptomatic before becoming symptomatic and then potentially infecting others.

In closing, the fact that SARS-CoV-2 is often asymptomatic led to a fundamental misunderstanding and miscommunication about its threat. Even if asymptomatic infections are commonplace, those relatively mild or benign outcomes can nonetheless lead to new infections that may be severe. When asymptomatic outcomes are invariably the norm, then the disease may end up being mild. When symptomatic outcomes are invariably the norm—and transmission is linked to symptoms—then it can be possible for us to use symptom-based behavior change both to avoid infecting others and to avoid becoming infected. But, for COVID-19, the amount of asymptomatic transmission lies somewhere in the middle for the population as a whole, even as the risk of asymptomatic transmission changed significantly with age. The collective consequence is that people's perceptions differed, and their behaviors were not necessarily linked to symptoms but to their perception of risk. Because mild and asymptomatic infections were common, misinformation and disinformation gained a foothold and flourished. This led to differences in behavior that could reduce spread. Ultimately, people who were asymptomatically infected became silent links in growing chains that led to more than 1 million deaths in the United States alone.

In total, both the outcome and the reasons for COVID-19's devastating impact represent a failure to confront asymptomatic transmission. But, amid the loss, there were programs and initiatives that helped to make things better. Some of these programs were local in scope, such as university testing initiatives. Other information tools had a wider reach that filled in the gaps and brought real-time information on risk to the public. Some programs grew more efficient over time, such as the commonplace use of rapid testing and improved ventilation. Still others became truly national and lifesaving in scope, including the development and distribution of vaccines to more than 100 million Americans within two years of the virus first being identified.

Assessing how to fight back and extend successes already in place while prioritizing investment in effective and often underutilized approaches is precisely the goal of the second part of this book.

PART II

PREPARING FOR PANDEMICS TO COME

CHAPTER 4

Respecting the Public

Put the Data into Their Hands

The Fog of Outbreak

At the start of March 2020, the COVID-19 pandemic remained largely an abstraction in much of the world. The number of documented cases remained low. Yet there was a sense of inevitability of the dangers to come. Reports out of Wuhan from January 2020 suggested that COVID-19 could spread rapidly from person to person and had a significant fatality rate, on the order of 1–2% overall, with risk of severe disease increasing substantially with age. The *Diamond Princess* cruise ship departing from Hong Kong had been quarantined in early February 2020 after hundreds of passengers had become infected—ultimately, more than a dozen individuals on this cruise died as a result of infections. By late February, parts of northern Italy in the Lombardy region were in complete lockdown because of the rapidly spreading infection. In the United States, March 2020 began without a single stay-at-home order. For the public, action-taking might have seemed premature. As of March 1, 2020, there were only 42 documented cases and 8 documented fatalities in the entire United States, largely concentrated near Seattle.[1] But these numbers belied a hidden and rapidly growing problem on a national scale.

COVID-19 has been exceptionally hard to stop for many reasons, but the central reason is that, for some, a COVID-19 infection leads to symptomatic disease, which can progress rapidly to severe disease, hospitalization, intubation, and death. In contrast, for many individuals, especially younger people, an infection need not translate into symptomatic illness. Instead, averaging over different age groups, approximately 50% of infections may be "asymptomatic"—that is, individuals are likely to "feel fine" and have mild, nonspecific, or subclinical symptoms. Yet, feeling fine or well enough to leave home may actually worsen pandemic severity at the population scale (as explained in part 1). In the first months of 2020, it was evident that SARS-CoV-2 could transmit asymptomatically, although the importance of such transmission remained uncertain.[2]

That was about to change.

As a result of an information vacuum in early 2020, many scientists working in epidemic (and adjacent) fields began to turn to social media, and Twitter in particular,[3] to try and communicate the expanding threat far beyond the confines of conventional academic debates. Richard Lenski, an elected member of the National Academy of Sciences and professor of microbiology at Michigan State University, began to refocus his small but influential blog on COVID-19 news and the potential risk for devastating spread. His central point was that the particular epidemiological mechanisms of COVID-19 could generate risks well beyond those anticipated from case counts alone. Lenski encouraged those who read his blog to prepare for the possibility that the United States would experience an even worse outbreak than had taken place in China. Lenski even took the preemptive step of shutting down his laboratory on March 9, 2020, including a temporary suspension of a world-recognized, long-term experiment on the evolution of bacterial lineages.[4] He did so to protect both the people working in his lab while taking the necessary steps to preserve key experiments. His message on March 9 was simple:

> Hopefully, some future historian of science will look back on today's entry and say: "What the hell was that all about?"[5]

If only that were so.

The threat highlighted by Lenski was reinforced by real-time analysis by Richard Neher (a professor at the Biozentrum at the University of Basel, Switzerland)—who cautioned in early February 2020 of the dangers in misinterpreting what seemed like low, perhaps even inconsequentially low, case count data. Neher is the codeveloper of Nextstrain. Nextstrain aggregates viral sequence data and places it into an evolutionary and geographic context days or even hours after sample analysis is complete.[6] The Nextstrain site is jointly led by a coalition of scientists and engineers, including Neher as well as Trevor Bedford (of the Fred Hutchinson Cancer Center of Seattle, also known as The Hutch), James Hadfield (of The Hutch), Emma Hodcroft (of the University of Basel in Switzerland), and many more evolutionary biologists, virologists, and software engineers. Neher offered the following take in a February 9, 2020, tweet:

> Simply put, many places might just be 2–3 months behind Wuhan and a variable rate of spread might result in a protracted pandemic with ups and downs. This is not a given, but overinterpreting the current case counts can be very misleading.[7]

A total of 26 people "liked" the tweet. In effect, insights by thoughtful scientists were being lost in the void. Indeed, the next day—on February 10, 2020—Trevor Bedford had discussed the evidence for human-to-human transmission found in viral genomes as part of a SARS-CoV-2 rapid response forum held at Georgia Tech. I organized and spoke at this forum on the dangers of epidemic spread in light of early estimates of its epidemiological features.[8] At the time, working with Sang Woo Park of Princeton University, Jonathan Dushoff of McMaster University, and epidemiology colleagues, we had already developed some of the earliest aggregate estimates of the basic reproduction number for COVID-19. Our estimate was that the basic reproduction number (R_0) of COVID-19 was close to 3. This meant that we should prepare for rapid case growth and potentially large population-level infections and consequences. The third speaker, Phil Santangelo, a professor of biomedical engineering at Georgia

Tech, discussed the potential for development of RNA-based vaccines and the pressures to begin to pursue solutions even at this early stage. Indeed, the race to develop scalable vaccines was already well underway.[9,10,11]

In early February 2020, our rapid response forum remained a niche event. It drew a standing-room-only crowd of scientists and engineers who came to hear talks by specialists intended to provide a glimpse into three critical themes of pandemic response: genomic surveillance, epidemiological modeling, and vaccine development. Notably, a lunch buffet was served. It would be a long time before such events were allowed back on the Georgia Tech campus.

Trevor Bedford was one of the earliest in the US scientific community to recognize the SARS-CoV-2 threat. He had been monitoring reports of a cluster of influenza-like illnesses and associated genetic sequences from Wuhan. The viral genomes had all the indicators of being closely related to one another. Worse, they shared the same set of mutations relative to that of the ancestral strain. This was a hallmark sign that the virus had passed from human to human rather than independently from some environmental, zoonotic reservoir. This was significant and disturbing. It meant that humans did not need to be in contact with an animal in a zoonotic reservoir (whether bat or pangolin) to become infected. Instead, the disease was now spreading human to human—often cryptically[12]—such that specific combinations of mutations found in an infector could be found in viruses within individuals they infected. And, if we could spread SARS-CoV-2 to each other, this meant that containment needed to be implemented rapidly—if it wasn't already too late.

Bedford and other virologists quickly leveraged genetic findings to accelerate the development of mRNA vaccines. This work required identifying key parts of the viral genome that could serve as a template for sending messages to train the human immune system to recognize the spike protein before the actual virus showed up.[13] Bedford's message, delivered by videoconference to those on the Atlanta campus, was simple: COVID-19 could spread rapidly, it could spread cryptically, and it was of significant threat to the United States.

The evidence was becoming clear. One individual could easily infect others.[14] Many of the infections were asymptomatic. Many individuals who were infected did not know they were infected and could easily infect others unwittingly. Crucially, it was quite likely that nearly every single human on the planet was immunologically naive—and vulnerable to infection.

Between March 8–10, coincident with the Skagit Valley Chorale rehearsal (as described in chapter 2), and after having spent the past six weeks analyzing the potential for symptomatic and asymptomatic spread using mathematical models linked to early case data, I posted on my Twitter account a series of warnings about the growing dangers associated with gatherings. By March 10, I consolidated my central message with the following warning:

> For organizers of large events, please consider the following: increases in #COVID19 cases means that soon (if not already), the chances of a positive case amongst a large pool of attendees (with all the consequences thereof) comes with increasing risk.[15,16]

The warning was accompanied with a graphic (figure 4.1).

This graph was seen by hundreds of thousands of Twitter users in the space of a few days, and many more times that number viewed the graph as it began to circulate and spread. It had become a "viral tweet."[17] The message had gotten through and was spreading outward quickly, given the connection between data, risk, and real-life events. Of course, a few hundred, a few thousand, or even a few million Twitter users is a pebble's worth of impact in a much larger sea. One million impressions is the likely reach of anything a pop star says or does or tweets about, even the most mundane of topics—the taste of a morning coffee—to say nothing of a new selfie or album that will be viewed millions, if not many tens of millions, of times. But, for scientists, whose work is typically read by a handful of experts, whether in the peer-reviewed literature or an otherwise bland professionally centered social media account, this depiction had clearly resonated beyond the confines of normal academic work. The graphical depiction of risk resonated because it put information into terms that allowed individuals

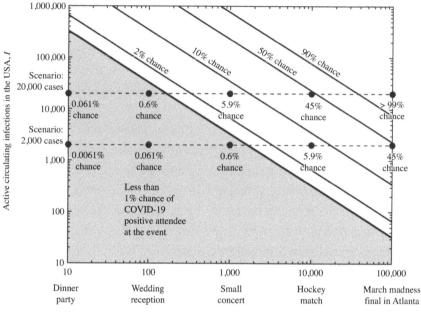

Note: Risk is $\epsilon \approx 1 - (1 - p_I)^n$ where $p_I = I / (330 \times 10^6)$ and n is event size.

Figure 4.1. COVID-19 Event Risk Assessment Planning Tool's graphical depiction of potential risk associated with attending events of different sizes, according to different levels of circulating infections in the United States. Estimates are of the chance that one or more individuals are positive for COVID-19 at an event, given its size and the current case prevalence. The model uses a binomial function to connect event sizes (on the x-axis) with the number of circulating cases (on the y-axis). *Source*: Weitz, J.S. (2020). COVID-19 event risk assessment planner. Figshare. https://doi.org/10.6084/m9.figshare.11965533.v1. Licensed under Creative Commons CC BY 4.0 DEED Attribution 4.0 International. https://creativecommons.org /licenses/by/4.0/.

to take their health into their own hands, even in the absence of public health decisions on event size restrictions or stay-at-home orders.

Indeed, the analysis was not spurred by an ongoing debate in the scientific literature. The analysis was spurred by a friend's question: Should he go to an upcoming Atlanta United soccer game? What was the risk that he and his family might be exposed and infected?

The challenge in answering that question was that the data remained unclear, enough so to generate a false sense of security. Asymptomatic infections and under-testing meant that there were many times fewer documented cases than actual infections. If one were to use the documented case counts alone, then it would seem implausible that events at that time should pose much risk—even large events. Likewise, if one were to think that asymptomatic cases were nearly a 100 times higher, then the epidemic did not merit the issuance of grave public health warnings (see part 1 on the fallacy of the COVID-19 comparison to seasonal influenza). There was also the problem of communication. Would informing individuals of the potential risk really change behavior in practice? In other words, what did it matter if there were 200 infections or 2,000 or even 20,000 in the entire United States, which has a population of approximate 330 million. For most people, it was easy enough to rationalize those 20,000 cases as being located far, far away, in a town or state completely disconnected from one's own life. As a result, reporting total cases in the United States or even cases per 100,000 (as has become the norm) are the kinds of information that may be useful to experts but glide off the surface of intuition to those who have limited time to parse pandemic news. The numbers become meaningless signifiers of expertise and of precision, changing little in practice.

The challenge was that numbers cannot tell their own story. But, numbers can act as a sail to drive a narrative forward.

Risk Models and Communication

What were the odds that my friend and his family might be exposed to COVID-19 at a professional soccer match held indoors? What are the odds that someone—perhaps **you**—might be exposed to COVID-19 at an indoor event or gathering? These were (and remain) the sort of questions that have become the most relevant and most difficult to answer—not just in early 2020 but multiple years later. The challenge is that answering such questions requires reasoning through a sequence of chance events, weighing the potential that the unlikely event might in fact happen.

A transmission event requires that someone is infected nearby and may potentially expose others. Then, they would have to be close enough to others to transmit—for example, by sharing air. Such risks are elevated at large events at concession stands, in bathrooms, hall-ways, lines, the stands, or anywhere individuals are crowded together indoors. If someone were to show up asymptomatically infected at an event, then they would almost certainly have no idea they were infected, and they would be more likely to infect one other person or perhaps even many others. At the time, indoor mask-wearing was nearly nonexistent for the majority of those living in Atlanta (and nationwide). Hence, by turning the question around, perhaps it might be possible to estimate and communicate a meaningful feature of transmission risk.

The objective of the graph was to inform and warn the public of the potential risks of transmission associated with large gatherings, even as there appeared to be little to no risk of infection in light of the relatively small number of *documented* SARS-CoV-2 cases. There were, as of March 10, 2020, only 1,500 cumulative cases in the entire United States. There are ~330 million people in the United States. Given the gap, why bother to worry about standing or sitting next to one of just a very small number of individuals with active infections—especially if individuals had symptoms and were likely to stay home if infected? Yet, case counts were almost certainly significant underestimates of infection burden for multiple reasons.

First, the commonplace nature of asymptomatic infections meant that many individuals were unlikely to be cognizant of having been infected and therefore unlikely to stay at home or seek testing. Second, testing was extremely limited, even for symptomatic individuals. Third, the number of documented fatalities already suggested that actual cases must be far higher and that SARS-CoV-2 was spreading rapidly in the background. There had been 23 reported fatalities in the United States between March 3 and March 10. These individuals presumably had been infected about 3 weeks earlier (in light of time-course data already available out of Wuhan). If the infection fatality rate was approximately 1%, then there should have been ~2,300 actual cases approximately 3 weeks beforehand. Yet there had been only 2 documented cases between February 12 and February 19 in the United States. Even with improvements in reporting, it seemed likely that underestimates by factors of 10 to 20 were appropriate. If so, then many individuals might feel fine even while unwittingly shedding virus and transmitting to others—an issue compounded by gatherings and events, where the virus could jump between otherwise disconnected groups and ultimately between cities, counties, and states. Given that individuals can shed virus for approximately 10 days and in some cases up to 14 days after infection (the rationale for extending isolation for 2 weeks), then the observation of ~1,500 new cases between March 1 and March 10, 2020, suggested that 15,000 individuals might be currently infectious (assuming a 10:1 documented to actual case ratio) or even 30,000 (assuming a 20:1 documented to actual case ratio).

In order to connect the number of documented cases to the risk of potential exposure and transmission at events, consider a scenario where there were 3,000 circulating cases in the entire United States. This is equivalent to a per capita infection rate of 1 in 100,000 individuals. Alternatively, if 30,000 were infected, that is equivalent to a per capita infection rate of 1 in 10,000 individuals. These two scenarios were far more likely than per capita infection rates estimated by raw documented case counts alone. At such levels, the probability that someone in an event is infected rapidly increases. But still, how does one connect circulating cases in the United States at large to the risk that someone might be infected at a particular event of a particular size?

The risk can be estimated by using a direct analogy to finding a bad penny in a pile. Imagine that someone has placed a small number of bad pennies amid a very large pile of good ones. If you were to grab 50 pennies at random, what are the chances that you have unwittingly selected a batch with one (or more) bad pennies? Imagine the case in which 1 in 100 pennies are bad. In that case, there is a 99% chance that the first penny is good; likewise, there is a 99% chance the second penny chosen is good, and so on. Hence, the chance that all the pennies are good is the product of $0.99 \times 0.99 \times \ldots \times 0.99$ (50 times over). If that is the chance that all the pennies are good, then the chance that one is bad is 1 minus 0.99 raised to the 50th power. Do you have an intuition or feel for the answer to this probability? For most of us, the answer is no, of course not. Nor should you. In this case, the actual odds are approximately 40% that someone will have taken a batch with a bad penny, even though bad pennies are very rare. The same type of probability calculation means that even if the odds of a bad penny were 1 in 1,000, there would still be a 5% chance that a randomly selected batch of 50 pennies would contain at least one bad one. In pandemic terms, those odds could easily lead to bad outcomes—because that one person in a crowd unaware of the risk is likely to infect many others, just as happened in the Skagit Valley Chorale practice.[18]

Hence, rather than asking individuals to take the per capita probability of infection and then embark on mental gymnastics leading nowhere, the graph that I shared on Twitter combined three principles together:

1. *Connect to real-life situations.* The graph (figure 4.1) explicitly includes a series of event sizes and connected them to the kinds of events that individuals might attend. The choice of words— dinner party, wedding reception, small concert, hockey match (or game), and March Madness—helped to explore event sizes by successive factors of 10.

2. *Do not let uncertainty generate an information vacuum.* Plausible ranges were used for the number of circulating infections as a means to estimate the value of the per capita infection rate without ever communicating the probability directly. This allowed reported numbers (on the y-axis) to remain in meaningful terms—circulating infections—even if the exact number of circulating infections was impossible to estimate precisely.

3. *Present numbers that matter.* The graphic depicted the results of the risk calculation by showing contour lines—that is, combinations of event sizes and case levels that would lead to the same chance that one or more individuals might be infected in an event of that size. As is apparent, if cases were significantly underestimated, then even relatively small events (like a chorus rehearsal) were likely to become potential superspreading events. Moreover, large events were already very likely to become the basis for rapid spread.

The rapid increase in risk suggested that even in scenarios with less than 1 case per 10,000 individuals nationwide, there would still be a coin-flip chance that one or more individuals might show up to March Madness infected. And March Madness was meant to culminate with a Final Four with an estimated crowd of more than 80,000 watching games together at Mercedes-Benz Stadium in Atlanta.

Instead, the National Collegiate Athletic Association (NCAA) canceled March Madness on March 12, 2020.[19]

There is another point worth learning from this small, bespoke graph on the risk of SARS-CoV-2 transmission associated with events of different sizes. This kind of quantitative estimate was released directly on social media, bypassing conventional routes of academic communication in order to address the vacuum generated by uncertainty. The graph and message would have taken weeks, if not months, to be published in a conventional academic journal using the standard approach to peer review. A paper on this ideal alone would almost certainly have been rejected. There was little mathematical novelty to the idea. Moreover, there was uncertainty. Yet precisely because of that uncertainty, it was critical to provide multiple options (i.e., scenarios in the graph). Even worse—from an academic perspective—the message had relevance in a particular moment in time. The time would change. The particular contour lines and assumptions would become outdated. Many scientists were facing the same challenge. How does one meaningfully bring quantitative toolsets to aid in a public health crisis when academic work and reward systems were set up for altogether different timescales? It seemed as if a very different approach was necessary. That approach must be able to differentiate between problems that required the laborious process of peer review as the apex of scientific discourse and problems that required a fundamentally direct dialogue—between scientists and the public.

This tension, and one way to address it, is the topic of the next section.

Building Pandemic Communication Platforms

How does one communicate to tens if not hundreds of millions worldwide that something bad may be about to happen—and that wholesale changes are needed in the fundamental way in which we live and work? These questions might seem the work of academics in concept, but they are the work of governments and public health organizations in practice. Virality aside, institutional actors have ready-made mechanisms, communications offices, connections to media, and operations teams that have training, experience, and resources to act as translators in a moment of crisis. In the United States, the Centers for Disease Control and Prevention (CDC) and state health organizations ostensibly had the kind of infrastructure needed to facilitate direct dialogue between science, scientists, and the public. Globally, the World Health Organization (WHO) ostensibly had the expertise and experience to become the preeminent source of information on the emerging pandemic. But COVID-19 has revealed fundamental inadequacies in the link between rigorous epidemic research, the assessment of uncertainty, and the communication of accurate information to the public at large.

In essence, for many countries—particularly the United States—the problem was too big and moving too fast, and conventional public health organizations (including the WHO and CDC) were too slow, often ill-equipped, and often organized around communicating with restraint until uncertainties were resolved.[20,21,22] Such approaches may work well when fighting established chronic or infectious diseases, but they are poorly suited to face a dynamic battlefield with uncertainty. There was always going to be uncertainty when facing an emerging infectious disease. As such, reliance on the default message that we are not yet sure, or overreliance on an inherent reticence to declare the obvious until scientifically proved beyond any doubt, ended up being a dangerous and defeating path. Disproving any doubt can take years. But actions were needed often weeks, if not days or even hours, after patterns of evidence came to light.

On top of all of these issues was a political challenge: the evidence often conflicted with the desired outcome for those responsible for disseminating key messages. This book is not one focused on politics— others are both more informed and better suited to discuss the spread of misinformation and other direct and indirect consequences of political failings and some successes, like Operation Warp Speed.[23] This book is meant to explain the science connecting the asymptomatic nature of spread to failures in stopping COVID as it emerged and to opportunities to improve the fight against pandemics to come. Hence, rather than address issues related to pandemic communication writ large, we will continue to use the asymptomatic nature of COVID-19 spread as a lens to explore one particular way in which it is possible to communicate, not just with a one-off Twitter thread, but with a sustained risk communication platform and campaign.

In doing so, consider the question paramount in spring and summer 2020: What is the risk of being exposed and infected? This period marked the loosening of restrictions in the United States, with policies varying significantly by state and partisanship.[24] (Although the USA's pandemic response may appear uniquely decentralized, similar tensions between economic and public health policymaking persisted globally.[25,26,27]) But opening up did not mean that the risk had been averted. In some cases, the rationale for relaxing a state's COVID-19–induced strictions was justified through misinterpretation of viral trends.[28]

The reopening of economies generated even more questions and new uncertainties as individuals—and not local, state, or national governments—decided how to respond. The commonplace nature of asymptomatic transmission meant that a mundane choice to go to a dinner party, to visit friends, to enter a store (mask on or mask off), to open the door to a family member or delivery driver, to go to work, or to sit on a bus or subway car were each infused with uncertainty and threat. How was one to be sure that someone else in that crowd was not infected? In fact, one could not be sure. The challenge of a disease that presents itself as asymptomatic in approximately 50% of infections and that has significant presymptomatic transmission means that absolute certainty regarding risk is the last thing anyone could offer. But, surely, it should be possible for individuals to have access to real-time information on the odds—or risk—that someone near them might be infected so that they can take charge of their own behavior and, by extension, their own health.

Let us therefore revisit the example described in the previous section, but rather than focus on a singular moment in time, we will pose the question: How can one continue to deliver estimates of risk associated with events of different sizes in a sustainable pandemic communication platform? The answer is that to build real-term analysis platforms of use to the public, scientists need to take a different approach to scientific work and communication. They cannot remain in their laboratories or on their computers if they want to make an impact. Nor can they communicate alone. As we will see, successful tools rely on interdisciplinary collaborations because different skill sets and expertise are required both behind the scenes and in front of the public.[29] Building up such tools has all the hallmarks of a startup environment, with the end product being the kind of creative act that can then be ported into institutional practice and cultures.

The images in the viral graphic shown in figure 4.1 combine a statistical model of risk with key pieces of information: (i) the number of documented cases, (ii) estimates on the extent to which infections are underreported, and (iii) the typical duration of infections. These three elements can be combined together to estimate what is termed *prevalence* (i.e., the fraction of the population that is infected at any given moment in time). If the duration of an infection is approximately 10 days (irrespective of symptoms), and if one knew the cumulative number of individuals infected over the past 10 days, then it would be possible to add these up as a rough estimate of the number of individuals who are infected now (i.e., they would almost certainly show up positive in a PCR test). In that 10-day period, it is likely that individuals may only be infected for a portion of the time (e.g., half that period). Nonetheless, in the interest of caution, we took the step of adding up cases over the past 10 days and then multiplying the documented cases reported by state agencies by an "ascertainment bias"—for example, 10 actual infections for each reported case and then later, as testing improved, biases that were centered closer to a 5:1 ratio.

Yet, it was also clear that producing a single graphic for the United States would also be problematic over the long term. All pandemics are local—even global pandemics like COVID-19. That is, the pandemic experience differs for someone in a rural county in Georgia as compared to someone in Seattle or New York or in the Mountain West outside of Denver. The disease may be the same, but the timing of arrival of cases, the intensity of spread, the density of interactions, and even the age demographics will differ, such that it is misguided to offer a single risk level to a country as large and diverse as the United States. Hence, it was essential to take the national-level risk contours in that viral tweet and connect them to local experiences.

In doing so, an expert in geographic spread and geographic information systems (GIS) was needed. Thankfully, I was already working with such an expert: Clio Andris, now associate professor of interactive computing as well as urban and regional planning at Georgia Tech. Andris is well known for her work on GIS data and networked systems, the kinds of systems in which interactions move along corridors and links.[30] As a result, much of her work focuses on placing interactions in a map context, often because interactions are driven by social or geographic ties that themselves represent a narrower set of interactions than are possible in a community. Clio and I had been working together on how to improve the dissemination of analytics tools for the public good—albeit in an entirely different topic area. But, when COVID-19 hit, we started to discuss a convergence of our skills: estimating and communicating risk at the level where action-taking is most likely—that is, not just national- or state-level estimates, but at the level of counties.

The resulting product—the COVID-19 Event Risk Assessment Planning Tool—was released on July 7, 2020.[31] It was codeveloped by our two groups along with the technical skills of a software engineering team spun out of Georgia Tech. What happened? The website (https://covid19risk.biosci.gatech.edu) crashed on the very first day. This was a good and a bad sign. The good news was that the crash was a result of overuse. We had tens of thousands of visitors per hour soon after launch. The bad news was that our team had to work to harden the underlying server system given two constraints:

1. We had no money to buy software or new computers.
2. We had a day to fix the problems.

Thankfully, we had a few key assets on our side—a remarkably talented team of volunteer software engineers and full stack developers founded by Georgia Tech graduates at the Applied Bioinformatics Laboratory (in particular, Aroon Chande and later Lavanya Rishishwar); the support of a talented early-career GIS student (Seohla Lee); and a deeply experienced colleague in the scientific computing architecture division at Georgia Tech (Troy Hilley). Together, the software engineers figured out that we could take a free version of the RShiny software package and deploy a server that managed the incoming visitor load across many parallel implementations of the same website being run on virtual machines.[32] The net result was that we could accommodate tens of thousands a visitors at the same time. And they came. Not just tens of thousands but hundreds of thousands in a single day. In one week, this academic website that provided risk maps at the county level and allowed users to change the event size to evaluate risks associated with different events had provided more than 1 million localized estimates. This was direct scientist-to-public communication, and it was working. Figure 4.2 is a black-and-white snapshot of the earliest risk assessment maps, taken from August 1, 2020, soon after the site was launched. As is apparent, the risk is not the same everywhere, which is a hallmark of a disease whose spread was highly structured as it moved across different regions in the United States.

This kind of website provided a real-time estimate of risk that one or more individuals might be infected in events of different sizes. It allowed users to zoom in and out at the county level, to change the event size, and to explore the role of underreporting with a slider that selected among plausible underreporting levels. In doing so, the website had a series of informational tips on how to reduce risk (e.g., avoid events, wear a mask, improve ventilation, or meet outdoors).

A local real-time approach has multiple advantages. The map-based presentation obviates the need to battle with interpreting the kinds of technical contour lines shown in figure 4.1. Moreover, the map can be updated automatically, every day, using publicly available data combined with a built-in statistical estimator. The website can scale to meet increasing access, and indeed, the access did fluctuate in intensity,

Date: August 1st, 2020   Ascertainment bias = 5

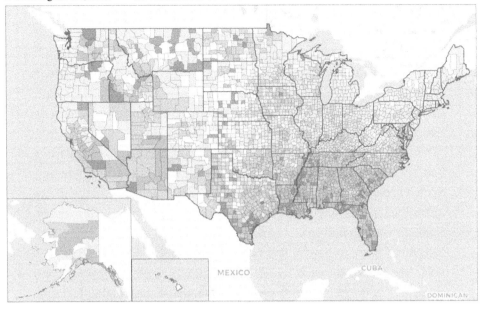

Figure 4.2. COVID-19 Event Risk Assessment Planning Tool's map of risk associated with events of size 50 (i.e., 50 people present), using an ascertainment bias of 5:1 per reported case. Darker counties represent a higher risk of cases. The online tool included a color-based range of risk, a risk legend, and additional information on interpretation and action-taking to prevent infections. *Source*: Adapted from figure 1 of Chande, A., et al. (2020). Real-time, interactive website for US-county-level COVID-19 event risk assessment. *Nature Human Behaviour* 4: 1313–1319. https://doi.org/10.1038/s41562-020-01000-9.

often increasing in direct proportion to the intensity of spread. But, since spread varied, it was apparent that individuals from different regions would find the site at different moments, spurred not only by word-of-mouth and social media but also by the appearance of the website on nightly news and print media sources. Since launch of the county-level map on July 7, 2020, and before being placed into archival mode in early 2023, the website was visited by more than 16 million unique individuals, including by individuals in every state, and provided more than 60 million risk estimates to the public at large. The website was featured in hundreds of media outlets (including the *Washington Post*, *LA Times*, *New York Times*, the BBC, National Geographic, CNN, and beyond), and the peer-reviewed article in *Nature Human Behaviour* was ranked more influential than >99.9% of nearly 400,000 scientific articles published in 2020 as ranked by their online attention by the Altmetric site (an evaluator of real-time impact of scientific articles).[33] Yet, the vast majority of the public in the United States never visited the site. Indeed, the collective impact represents only a partial scope of the opportunity to nowcast risk, if leveraged and included as part of national-level investment.

Imagine, if such risk estimates driven by asymptomatic transmission had been available on mobile apps from the outset of the pandemic. Such a scenario is not implausible, given what a small group of committed scientists and engineers, volunteering their time on top of funded research and teaching duties, was able to do on short notice. Imagine if such estimates had been disseminated as part of CDC reports and White House briefings and communicated in simple graphics as part of evening news broadcasts (alongside the weather report). All of this could have been possible in place of misleading and cherry-picked model results (as already reviewed in chapter 1). The science was there, as was the technology. Individuals should have been able to make an informed choice. Given real-time information, they could have decided based on their personal health situation if the risk was worth bearing. With information, perhaps they could have decided that they would be better off missing an event.

Of course, many individuals had no such option.

Pandemic response policies did not provide the economic safeguards to ensure that individuals could hold on to their jobs or work in distinct modes—those on the front line of health responses were at least aware of these risks, and in many cases they were able to wear the kind of preventative masks that could save their lives. Yet for others working in food-service industries, in eldercare, or in first-responder jobs, these kinds of risk maps could potentially inform an individual's choice to wear a high-quality mask or to advocate for better protections.[34] These risk maps also had the potential to help decision-makers in the public health arena and private sector invest in the kinds of simple, low-cost approaches to improve ventilation in work sites and reduce risk. Some of these steps have been taken, but not enough.

And yet, before switching to the kind of sustainable risk communication needed to fight the next pandemic, it is important to ask: Do we have evidence that this risk communication is effective? What does it matter if individuals know the risk of exposure if there is nothing they can do about it, or perhaps worse, if individuals know the risk but simply do not care?

Measuring the Power of Information

In early 2021, soon after the publication of a peer-reviewed article describing the COVID-19 Event Risk Assessment Planning Tool, our team at Georgia Tech was contacted by Allie Sinclair. Sinclair was a PhD student in cognitive neuroscience at Duke University working with faculty members Gregory Samanez-Larken and Alison Adcock on problems related to awareness, risk perception, and behavior change (Sinclair has since completed her PhD dissertation work and is now a postdoctoral scientist at the University of Pennsylvania). It had been apparent since early 2020 that changes in behavior had strong impacts on the overall changes in pandemic dynamics—for better and for worse. It was less clear whether or not it was possible to shift someone's behavior in periods or situations associated with elevated risks of infection. Public health campaigns can take a long time. Habituating commonsense practices can originate at the source (e.g., think of the municipal distribution of clean water) or through individual-centered action-taking (e.g., distributing free condoms on college campuses). Yet, for COVID, the asymptomatic mode of transmission meant that many were not even aware that they might be about to enter into a risky situation.

Sinclair and colleagues decided to put cognitive neuroscience-influenced interventions into practice. Working in 2020 and 2021, they asked volunteers to estimate the risk that one or more individuals had COVID-19 in an event of a certain size in their area (e.g., a coffee shop with 25 people, a restaurant with 50 people, or perhaps a retail store with 100 shoppers inside). Then, they used the COVID-19 Event Risk Assessment Planning Tool website that our team at Georgia Tech had developed as a means to compare the estimates of volunteers with current best-estimates of realized risk. The individuals volunteering in the study were then informed on the extent to which they were potentially overestimating or underestimating risk at a particular event. Finally, Sinclair and colleagues asked the volunteers to imagine that they were about to participate in that event again—and whether they were more or less willing to participate.

The results were striking. Receiving information from a reputable source, along with a visualization scenario of the risk involved, could help to potentially change the minds of those who underestimate the risk of participating in (typically) large, risky events.[35] This meant that as people became more aware of the underlying risk that one or more people at the event might be infected, they were then less likely to attend the event. Moreover, the results were particularly informative with respect to interventions for older adults. In that case, having older individuals visualize their risk helped them improve their understanding of risk and retain that perception for multiple weeks—suggesting that interventions could be impactful and durable.[36]

These promising results were done in a controlled study format with volunteers. Would similar results hold "in the wild"—that is, with individuals who visited the risk dashboard online?

Figure 4.3 is a black-and-white version of a still image from our revised COVID-19 risk website meant to test cognitive neuroscience interventions of risk-based visualizations and behavior change. Although the images appear simple, they represent more than six months of work by a team of Georgia Tech scientists, Duke cognitive psychologists, and software engineers from the Applied Bioinformatics Laboratory.

The work required translating principles of the controlled study into a format that was compatible with the layout, functioning, and feel of the risk site. It also required "human subjects approval"—that is, it needed authorization and review by both Georgia Tech and Duke

University's institutional review board to assess the ethics, suitability, and risks associated with asking questions of visitors to the website. In this case, the intervention was green-lighted by an expedited review process, as is typical for interventions that ask individuals to anonymously participate in an online quiz after consent. Yet, circling back to the premise of this chapter, even these expedited reviews, often shepherded by collaborative and competent institutional review board professionals, take a substantial amount of time. The proposal for approval of this intervention included more than 40 pages of documentation of the rationale, design, and implementation. All of this points to a genuine challenge: How does one get approval to intervene amid a public health crisis while balancing the real needs for suitable ethical review? In this case, the answer may have been simple, but streamlining this and other processes (e.g., laboratory approval for testing for SARS-CoV-2, as discussed in chapter 5) is essential for timely and meaningful public health interventions.

When it was deployed in October 2021 (coincidentally, just before the start of the Omicron wave), this intervention allowed visitors to the site to take a quiz and try out a visualization exercise after seeing the map. The focus of the study was to evaluate perceptions of risk *in the area of the individual visiting the site*, thereby connecting local perception of risk to individual estimates. After completing the quiz, individuals received an accuracy score, were shown the predicted risk, then asked if they were more or less willing to participate in events like the kind they had viewed.

Figure 4.4 summarizes the findings: such interventions can make a difference, whether information is presented by websites or by demographically balanced surveys.[37] Individuals in this study tended to overestimate the risk of small events and underestimate the risk of large events. When probed to reevaluate their behavior, visitors to the site indicated they were less willing to attend larger events (e.g., those with 25 to 1,000 people in attendance). This suggests that once individuals are informed of a gap in risk perception, they are willing to change their behavior, at least when it comes to certain types of gatherings. But there were caveats. People who overestimated risk did not show a greater

A

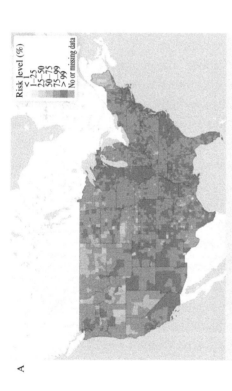

Risk level (%)
< 1
1–25
25–50
50–75
75–99
> 99
No or missing data

After viewing this map are you MORE or LESS
willing to participate in an event of this size?

Same as before

Much less   A little less   Same as   A little more   Much more
willing   willing   before   willing   willing

B   **Risk context**

You're *viewing* risk level for an event
with 50 people, which is like:

A supermarket

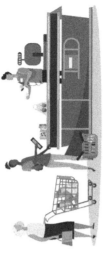

...or a restaurant

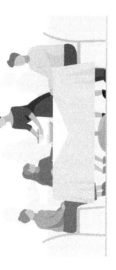

Figure 4.3. Visualization of the interactive elements developed as a means to assess the potential to leverage online dashboards to influence and potentially reduce high-risk behavior associated with COVID-19 transmission. *Source:* Sinclair, A.H., et al. (2023). Communicating COVID-19 exposure risk with an interactive website counteracts risk misestimation. *PLOS ONE* 18: e0290708. https://doi.org/10.1371/journal.pone.0290708

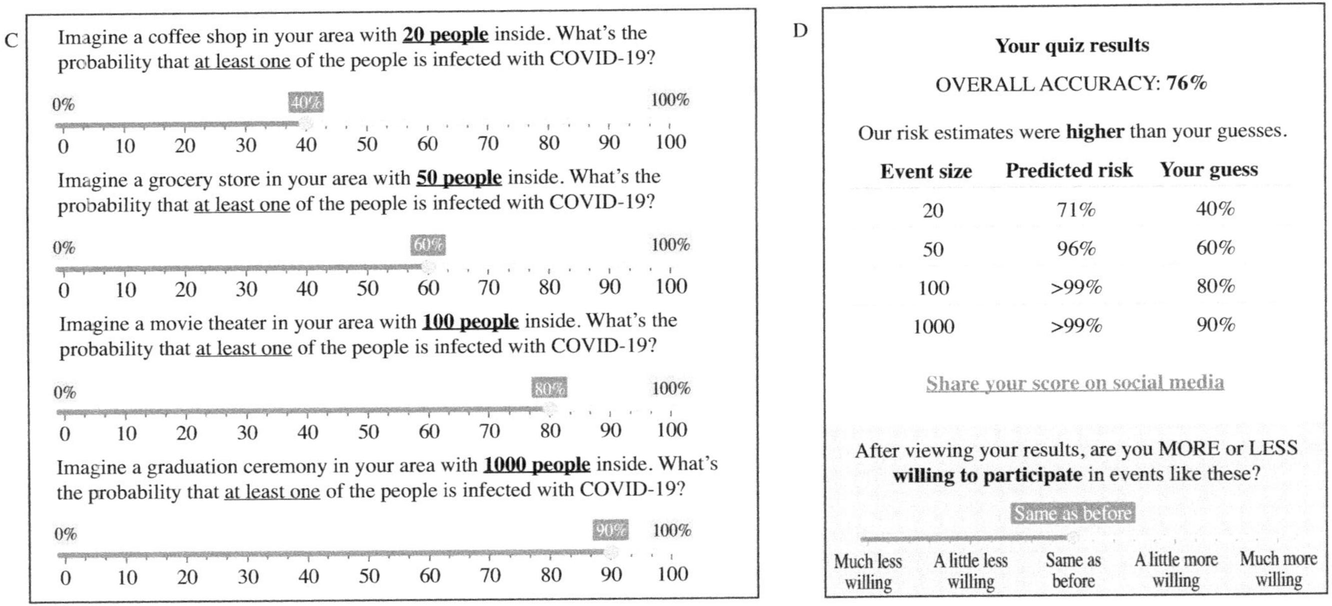

C

Imagine a coffee shop in your area with **20 people** inside. What's the probability that <u>at least one</u> of the people is infected with COVID-19?

0% |————[40%]————————————————————| 100%
0   10   20   30   40   50   60   70   80   90   100

Imagine a grocery store in your area with **50 people** inside. What's the probability that <u>at least one</u> of the people is infected with COVID-19?

0% |————————————[60%]————————————| 100%
0   10   20   30   40   50   60   70   80   90   100

Imagine a movie theater in your area with **100 people** inside. What's the probability that <u>at least one</u> of the people is infected with COVID-19?

0% |——————————————————————[80%]——| 100%
0   10   20   30   40   50   60   70   80   90   100

Imagine a graduation ceremony in your area with **1000 people** inside. What's the probability that <u>at least one</u> of the people is infected with COVID-19?

0% |——————————————————————————[90%]| 100%
0   10   20   30   40   50   60   70   80   90   100

D

Your quiz results

OVERALL ACCURACY: 76%

Our risk estimates were **higher** than your guesses.

Event size	Predicted risk	Your guess
20	71%	40%
50	96%	60%
100	>99%	80%
1000	>99%	90%

Share your score on social media

After viewing your results, are you MORE or LESS **willing to participate** in events like these?

Much less willing	A little less willing	Same as before	Same as before	A little more willing	Much more willing

Figure 4.3. continued

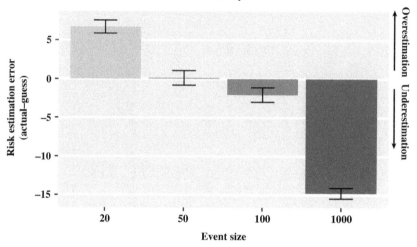

Risk misestimation by event size

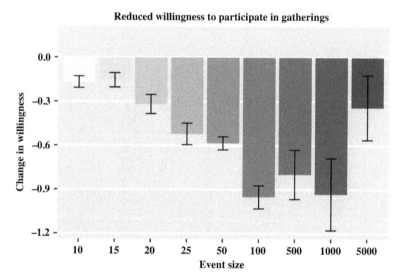

Reduced willingness to participate in gatherings

Figure 4.4. Risk misestimation and behavior change. One graph shows the estimation error in terms of the percentage gap between the website estimated risk and the participant's guess as a function of event size (upper panel). The other graph shows the change in willingness on a five-point scale in attending an event after an intervention (lower panel). A reduced willingness score of −1 denotes a shift from "a little less willing" to "a lot less willing." *Source*: Sinclair, A.H., et al. (2023). Communicating COVID-19 exposure risk with an interactive website counteracts risk misestimation. *PLOS ONE* 18: e0290708. https://doi.org/10.1371/journal.pone.0290708.

willingness to attend events. And there was no evidence that individuals were willing to change their behavior associated with smaller events. In other words, once you have committed to visit close friends and family, you are more likely to continue to make that choice irrespective of informed risk. These results provide a spectrum of public health relevant insights and provide hints as to why COVID-19 has been so hard to stop—and why far more targeted work is needed to make a long-term impact, whether for this pandemic or the next one.

Deciding on whether to attend a soccer match or even a concert is quite different from deciding to forgo a small social gathering, perhaps with family or one's closest friends. It is quite possible that improvements in public health communication—along with an improved focus on local risk estimation as a type of pandemic "nowcast"—could have helped reduce the frequency and size of superspreading events. Even if individuals decide to attend specific events knowing that there are almost certainly others in the crowd with COVID-19, there is still an opportunity for behavior change. Learning more about risk can be a motivation to change behavior during events (e.g., as evidenced by increased mask-wearing during the rest of 2020 and through the summer of 2021).

But not everybody wants to change their behavior. And, at some point, part of our objective should be to find ways to minimize pandemic impacts in the first place. The challenge in modifying behaviors at small events also suggests that communicating risk alone is a key step, but it is not the only step. It is essential to recognize that behavioral change will depend on whether one is faced with modifying something core or peripheral. Moreover, individuals can have vastly different risk tolerances. Over time, communicating and acknowledging objectives are keys to sustainable risk communication. When individuals do take the step to participate in events both small and large (as most of us now do regularly), then the onus must shift, in part, to institutions. Institutions must provide infrastructure to reduce the risk of asymptomatically infected individuals triggering a chain of events leading to severe infections or worse.

Action Opportunity: Reducing Transmission at Indoor Gatherings through Healthier Air, Targeted Masking, and Awareness Campaigns

Fighting back against COVID-19 requires a balance between doing the most epidemic good while doing the least socioeconomic harm. In that sense, the debate over lockdowns versus opening up represents a false dichotomy. There is not much prospect for a sustained socioeconomic recovery if individuals feel they are fundamentally unsafe when returning to work or school or going on holiday. Hence, choosing one or the other represents a limited imagination of what a sustained response could be. Part of the challenge of proposing alternative mitigation approaches is that if one only has blunt tools—like societal-scale lockdowns—then there is not much nuance left to develop and deploy strategically personalized approaches. But such personalized approaches are central to balance multiple objectives. To get them right, we must communicate the mechanisms most associated with transmission, who in fact is most at risk for severe cases, and then support interventions by bringing data-driven decision-making to institutions and individuals.

Asymptomatic transmission means that many individuals feel fine but can shed infectious virus, leading to a high risk of new transmission within indoor spaces with poor ventilation. The threat of indoor transmission should lead to a transformation of our approach to built environments—one that could come with both significant public health benefits.[38] It could also, with the right incentives, lead to significant economic development opportunities to design, retrofit, and build ventilation spaces that keep epidemic mitigation in mind—prioritizing air quality as much as water reuse and net energy use, as is the case with buildings certified according to leadership in energy and environmental design (LEED) standards.[39] The realities of asymptomatic transmission also means that certain contexts will continue to involve higher risks for individuals and that fundamental changes will be needed to selectively decrease risk of transmission. These risks may be due to larger-than-typical risks of spread in transit, involving high densities, crowded spaces, and extended time indoors—with meat-processing plants being one example.[40] These risks may also be due to larger-than-typical risks of severe outcomes in the event of transmission, an issue particularly relevant in hospital environments as well as in long-term care facilities.[41] Yet, even for all the concerted efforts of public health authorities to improve the ventilation landscape, the extent to which individuals tolerate or even embrace changes in behavioral norms requires that we share the rationale behind the choice. Information can change the behavior of trusted decision-makers, and the behavioral changes of those decision-makers can then drive subsequent changes in social groups who are likely to value social coherence even more so than individual adherence to public health mandates on the basis of the data or science alone.

The following short sections involve action items that could help to reduce respiratory disease transmission within the relevant context: indoor gatherings.

Upgrading the healthy air landscape

This book has described ways in which individuals can shed viruses through the air even when they feel fine. This may happen because they have a mild or asymptomatic infection or because their infection is initially asymptomatic and then becomes symptomatic over time. Either way, the absence of symptoms (or the absence of specific clinical symptoms) is not an indication of the absence of infectiousness. Obviously, testing can become a significant part of determining who is infected and when—a topic for the chapter 5. But testing was never meant to be a singular silver bullet. Indeed, multiple years of testing delays and logistical problems (including waits to get tested, get test results, and get help if positive), compounded by pricing structures that disincentivize testing or make testing infeasible, all suggest that testing must be a part, but not the only part, of the solution. As has been noted before, we can hope for the best—that individuals in an indoor gathering have tested negative recently—but realistically, this is unlikely to happen, and many would opt out even if large-scale tests were available.

This means that there must be a fundamental restructuring to preparing built environments in a way that anticipates that some individuals will be infected and breath out infectious viruses (COVID-19 and others) whenever groups congregate. How do we reduce the risk of events turning into spreading, and potentially superspreading, incidents and make it safer when groups do gather? A first step is to improve the quality of indoor air.

In light of pandemics, we can assess air quality in two primary ways: (i) whether or not the indoor air is "fresh"(i.e., as close as is possible to a healthy outdoor air environment) and (ii) whether or not the indoor air is relatively "sterile" (i.e., has low levels of viruses, bacteria, and mold). Getting there will require a mix of low-tech and high-tech solutions as well as shifts in social norms that foster individual and local engagement.

Breathing in fresh air requires, first of all, that the mix of oxygen and carbon dioxide in the air is similar to that outdoors. At present, carbon dioxide levels in the air are ~420 parts per million. (Interested readers can consult any number of climate change books to understand drivers of this environmental level over time.[42]) Yet, because individuals inhale oxygen and exhale carbon dioxide, the act of breathing can dilute the relative fraction of oxygen in the air while increasing the percentage of carbon dioxide. In a relatively short period of time, a poorly ventilated conference room filled with a dozen members of an office team can breathe out enough carbon dioxide so that levels rise more than 3-fold, to over 1,000 parts per million or even higher. Such levels would be catastrophic at global scales, but such levels in a conference room, classroom, retail store, or apartment are an indicator that the air turnover is insufficient.[43] Over short periods of time, individuals may get sleepy, make bad decisions, or start to breath in infectious viruses.[44] There is already a low-cost solution to measure indoor air quality: a carbon dioxide monitor. Such monitors can track the relative fraction of carbon dioxide (CO_2) in real time.[45] They should also be triggers for change.

One option would be to use CO_2 monitors as a trigger to open a window. Unfortunately, such a well-meaning policy would likely lead to yo-yo behavior and eventually complacency and a return to the poor baseline. Individuals would breathe out, collectively triggering a critical level of CO_2, and then someone (perhaps) would open a window for a short time so that the CO_2 level drops back, either just below the critical level or back to that of the outdoors. Yet, when the window closes in a poorly ventilated room, the CO_2 levels will climb upward again. In other cases, opening windows may not be feasible, such as on buses and trains and in many office buildings, places of work, hotels, and other multilevel dwellings. Addressing the freshness of air in these cases requires shifts in design standards for future-proofing the air of new construction while retrofitting and improving the standards of air circulation in existing buildings. Of course, environmental health and human health are fundamentally related. If buildings are designed to improve the circulation and exchange of indoor and outdoor air, yet the outdoor air has high levels of fine particulate matter—then an open window is hardly a safe alternative.

Fundamental redesigns of heating, ventilating, and air-conditioning (HVAC) systems will take time and investment, although thankfully, there are paths available now that can help to address indoor air quality before retrofitting buildings. Low-cost box filters can be installed and used in tandem to drive air through a fine mesh filter that is meant to capture particles while letting oxygen and carbon dioxide through. The use of such high-efficiency particulate air (HEPA) filters will not reduce CO_2 levels to that of the outdoors, but they will make air more sterile. One promising low-cost solution are so-called Corsi-Rosenthal boxes that include air entry and filtration through multiple HEPA filters connected to a box fan.[46] There are alternatives, including the use of upper-room ultraviolet C light (UVC) or heating elements. Caution is warranted in some cases. Certain disinfection approaches may inadvertently increase chemical pollutants by destabilizing particles, thereby changing the distribution of volatile aerosolized chemical compounds with potentially unexpected harms to human health.[47,48] By way of contrast, the widespread use of filters could become a norm to reduce the number of infectious virus particles—with many other side benefits as well in reducing the presence of bacteria and harmful mold and without the negative consequences of heat or UVC treatments. Detailed prescriptions for implementation are needed to expand "green" building design to include the impacts of air circulation systems on pathogen risk.

Targeted mask use in high-risk or high-spread environments

Before COVID-19, relatively few people in the United States used masks in public settings outside of hospital and medical environments. There were a few exceptions. Individuals accustomed to traveling in Asia would often wear masks in airports and transit hubs because the impact of SARS-1 and bird flu had already made mask wearing a social norm there.[49] In addition, individuals who were immunocompromised might sometimes make the same choice. The influenza pandemic of 1918–1919 sparked widespread adoption of masks in the United States, a practice that was replicated in the early phases of the COVID-19 pandemic, as detailed in part 1 of this book. Over time, mask-wearing shifted from being rare to commonplace practice (whether mandated or not), and then it transformed, to some extent, into a visual symbol of one's political views.[50] The sustainability of mask-wearing has limits. But there is a chance to use masks as part of a multilayered approach, especially if we leverage information on the spread of COVID-19 by individuals who are asymptomatic within indoor, poorly ventilated environments. In contrast, a nuanced mask policy especially in a post-vaccine society should also embrace an individual's right to decide whether to wear a mask, especially in those environments where risk is relatively low.

A combination of factors lead to increased risk of COVID-19 transmission. These factors include the number of individuals present, the setting (whether indoors or outdoors), and ventilation. These factors can also represent the basis for the use of targeted mask-wearing. One primary example is on buses and trains, where many individuals gather together, often in high densities for extended periods of times, and where it is often infeasible or impossible to open a window. These are the precise conditions that could (i) lead to the increased risk that one or more individuals are infected, (ii) increase the number of individuals exposed and infected, and (iii) make contact tracing and other means to track down sources of spread more difficult. If masking becomes commonplace or required (e.g., during periods of elevated spread), commuting environments will be critical in reducing transmission rates and dispersal of illness. Wearing masks is not a substitute for improved ventilation and air turnover, but it augments the response. The same principle applies to plane travel. Despite the benefits during boarding and deplaning procedures that bring many individuals in close contact, some people have strong negative reactions to mask-wearing, leading to conflicts with flight staff.[51] If we are to build a culture that actually uses masks in sensible ways, then we have to strive to identify those places where high-quality masks can make the most difference, clearly communicate the rules on their use, and then enforce the rules. If we are not willing to enforce rules and, instead, only "strongly" encourage mask-wearing, then we should not be surprised when levels of mask-wearing do not reach identified goals. In doing so, a few key principles must be kept in mind.

First, wearing masks outdoors as a means to prevent COVID-19 transmission is of limited value. Yes, there are exceptions, and there are many other reasons to wear a mask outdoors (e.g., sensitivity to allergies or to reduce intake of polluted air). But since the vast majority of documented infection has taken place indoors, then an impactful mask-wearing policy should focus on indoor environments. Likewise, if mask-wearing is required, then government partnerships will be necessary to provide appropriate masks in locations where they are required (e.g., in 2021, the Italian regional train system provided individually wrapped masks to passengers).

Second, mask-wearing some of the time in environments with indoor dining is of limited use. Hence, we have to decide if it is worth enforcing mask mandates when the context is one in which food is part and parcel of the experience. What value is it to have a mask requirement in a restaurant if the patrons remove their masks for extended periods of time to eat and drink? In such cases, even though restaurant patrons may wear a mask briefly at the front door or greeting station, they spend much more time without a mask, which makes the mask requirement less impactful in terms of public health outcomes. Moreover, encouraging mask-wearing only until one gets seated at a table also miscommunicates a fundamental reality of asymptomatic and airborne transmission. Individuals may mistakenly believe that once seated, the only people who could possibly infect them are the other patrons at the same table. This is not the case. The long-distance transmission in a restaurant in Guangzhou, China (first explored in chapter 2) demonstrated early in the pandemic that the six-foot rule was not in fact sufficient protection.[52] Instead, public health officials could honestly communicate the risk to patrons and staff and prioritize improved air circulation in indoor dining environments across the board: from fast-food chains to small, independent restaurants, college food courts, and dining facilities in long-term care facilities, while incentivizing the provisioning of outdoor options whenever possible. If Paris can do it, why not us?[53]

Third, we should consider the balance between risk of transmission and the chance that transmission will lead to severe outcomes in deciding when masks remain required—even if the majority of public spaces eventually become mask-free. For a salient example, consider nursing homes and long-term care (LTC) facilities. In the United States, more than 30% of COVID-19 fatalities in the first year of the pandemic were in such facilities, even though they accounted for a far smaller fraction of documented infections. Large-scale outbreaks were the norm, often including a substantial fraction of the residents and staff in a facility (sometimes half or more). As a result, these are the kinds of environments where mask-wearing by nonessential visitors and staff should become a standard moving forward. The use of mask-wearing by visitors, augmented potentially by rapid tests for visitors (to be revisited in the next section), can provide more layers of protection for deeply vulnerable communities. In doing so, the enforced use of masks—along with testing and increased ventilation—can help ensure that visits are in fact possible and that our grandparents and parents, relatives, friends, and colleagues can still feel the presence of loved ones. In doing so, more will also need to be asked of the investment made by certain LTC and nursing home operators to reduce the risk of spread in vulnerable communities.

Finally, any mask-wearing policy will have to address the divisiveness of mask policies in schools. Aggregate, comparative studies have shown that mask-wearing has an impact on the overall number of cases. In one case study from late 2020 in Georgia, adjacent school districts with mask mandates experienced nearly 40% fewer cases than those without mask mandates.[54] This example is bolstered by substantial evidence that masks can serve as a low-cost, community-wide strategy to contain and reduce the spread of SARS-CoV-2, both in the early stages[55] and later in the pandemic.[56] Yet, despite being a practical solution, mask-wearing in the United States remains a controversial,[57] politicized, and increasingly discarded policy,[58] outside of specialty settings.

There are many reasons for the move away from mask policy to individual choice.

Not everyone wears a mask properly, and because of intrinsic differences in attitudes, it is not uncommon to see people wearing a mask below their nose. Even when people are required to wear masks, they often take them off for lunch, when in crowded cafeterias or classrooms, or even during brief water or snack breaks. In an ideal world, if everyone wore a mask and ate outside, then the risk of school-based transmission could be significantly reduced. But such an ideal world takes a singular view of public health benefits, so instead we must acknowledge that the reasons for mandating masks have shifted. The risk of severe COVID-19 outcomes in children has, thus far, been comparable to that of influenza. Hence, from a public health perspective, reducing transmission broadly is important, but the primary aim of masking in schools is to avoid spreading the virus to older individuals (e.g., teachers and caregivers). Obviously, the challenges of protecting immunocompromised individuals are many.

Watchful monitoring of outcomes will continue to be important, but in the interim, it is likely that in practice, parents and children will give up on masks because (i) they (rightfully) perceive infections as being mild, (ii) rules are ambiguous and not enforced, and (iii) social pressures come into play. That is, in the absence of requirements, when they see that the people around them are not wearing masks, there can be a collective shift in attitude from situations where all are wearing masks to situations where no one is.[59] In the long-term, school leaders may decide to focus on disease outcomes rather than preventing transmission by leveraging existing vaccination policies that already authorize K–12 schools and colleges to mandate vaccines for many other diseases for students and staff.

Localized, real-time risk nowcasting (and forecasting)

The launch of the COVID-19 Event Risk Assessment Planning Tool on July 7, 2020, as a research website generated significant interest. Within the first days of launch, more than 500,000 individuals visited the site. In academic terms, that level of visitors is off the charts. In public terms, however, if that level of visitors were to continue for the year, it would imply that every American would have checked the risk of being exposed to COVID-19 in an event in their area just once every two years. In practice, the nearly "viral" level of visits did not continue at the same pace. Instead, interest fluctuated along with the risk of COVID-19, such that more than 16 million individuals visited the site in the first two years. That is approximately 16 million more individuals than who typically read an academic research paper. For our team, these numbers remained far beyond the largest reach of any academic project. By contrast, in conventional academic work, having a few thousand colleagues read an academic paper and a few hundred colleagues cite it represents a serious success. Therein lies a gap and an opportunity.

Why should real-time risk assessment have to bubble up from academic environments and remain there? Instead, what if the risk of COVID-19 exposure in a town, city, county, or region had been available every night, as easily accessible as the nightly weather reports, either on radio, TV, or the internet? What if such risk "nowcasting" or even short-term risk forecasting were part and parcel of basic communication platforms developed and disseminated throughout the United States? Rather than hearing a local government make a decision with respect to COVID-19 countermeasures in an information vacuum, efforts to localize and communicate risk in meaningful and accurate terms could become the gateway for public health decision-making as well as individualized responses. It is much harder to tell a community to wear masks when people perceive risks as decreasing and when their perceptions are shaped by social media echo chambers,[60] government officials who may use misleading information to implement public health responses,[61] and news headlines that provide a national and seemingly "psychologically distant" view of infection risk.[62]

Individuals should be able to know the risk that someone in a crowd or at an event may be infected. Such information can be estimated and has been estimable, albeit imperfectly since early 2020. The geotargeting of such risks requires links between datasets and communication platforms. The methodology remains simple enough that digital platforms should be developed that connect such risk communication platforms to a network of communicators that they may then select from, as if from a menu. Localized risk maps can be generated daily and shared as bulletins with long-term care facilities as part of welcome information that explains the rationale for why mask requirements are in place. Information on risk could be used in encouragement or requirement campaigns for wearing masks in targeted settings. Qualitative risk assessment could also be used to communicate and reinforce the importance of mask-wearing indoors, especially in locations where there is a high risk of transmission (public transit, schools, crowded work environments) or a high risk of severe outcomes from infection (long-term care facilities).

The COVID-19 Event Risk Assessment Planning Tool and the associated scientific publication was featured on hundreds of media outlets.[63] But the tool typically appeared just once, or perhaps a few times in a particular news market. That is because the tool stopped being news. Indeed, risk assessment tools are not meant to be breaking news; they are meant to function like weather reports. These tools can become a recurring feature that provides a barometer of values that individuals can use to make decisions regarding their individual health.

The government does not mandate the use of umbrellas when the weather forecaster says it will rain. If you decide not to carry an umbrella and get wet, that becomes your problem. But infectious diseases do not stop with you—they become a collective problem. As a result, it may be that the generation of such transmission risk reports could lead individuals to change their habits and opt to wear masks in specific circumstances, irrespective of risk. Older individuals or those who are immunocompromised may decide that being maskless on a bus, train, or plane is no longer tenable—especially in periods of high transmission—and they may systemically use one-way masking. Otherwise healthy, younger individuals may decide that their personal level of comfort with preventative measures will vary with risk. But pandemic fatigue is real and must be addressed to implement impactful programs that help avoid the crisis of large-scale transmission, hospitalization, and fatalities that was seen at multiple points from 2020 to 2022.

We cannot hope that a few academic researchers maintain what should be a large-scale initiative that could connect case and other infection data to real-time localized risk. For our part, our multidisciplinary team worked with the CDC to disseminate information on the risk of local infection. Many other academic groups have done the same. Long-term, stable support is required, however, to avoid burnout among those positioned to nimbly connect epidemic data to the public. The time to invest in such people and platforms is now—while keeping in mind that diversification of distributing funds is critical to ensure that creative ideas can flow from established and up-and-coming groups alike, rather than concentrating funds in a few research groups. If such support is in place, we may find new challenges and even have the opportunity to develop localized responses systems to curb outbreaks before they become globally devastating pandemics.

CHAPTER 5

Testing as a Form of Pandemic Mitigation

Doing More Testing, Finding More Cases

Why test at all? This question is legitimate, especially since testing has remained one of the most confusing and divisive components of the US pandemic response. The confusion started at the beginning, but perhaps it is best encapsulated by remarks from former president Donald Trump on May 14, 2020, in Allentown, Pennsylvania:

> We have more cases than anybody in the world. But why? Because we do more testing. When you test, you have a case. When you test, you find something is wrong with people. If we didn't do any testing we would have very few cases.[1]

At some level, such statements are akin to burying one's head in the sand, or worse. Not testing for cancer does not make the growing tumor disappear and can needlessly delay the potential for early treatments. The same holds for diseases like HIV, where testing can enable prompt retroviral treatment while also leading to changes in behavior that can protect sexual partners from exposure.[2] Yet, testing is not universally used as a means to control the spread of respiratory illnesses. Far from it. Society does not use PCR (polymerase chain reaction) viral testing for the common cold. It is possible that many tens of millions of people in the United States are infected with the common cold annually, whether caused by rhinoviruses or seasonal coronaviruses. But there is no way to know for certain. A doctor will not order a molecular viral test for the case of the sniffles. Why would they? What would change if the doctor or patient knew that information? Likewise, if COVID-19 was no more worrisome than seasonal influenza, or in some circles, no more to be feared than the common cold, then why should we test at all? Why not simply address symptoms and treat those who are sick? To answer the question of testing requires breaking down the potential value of testing, including its potential use as a form of mitigation.

Testing can serve multiple public health goals. For the individual and the physician, the usual purpose of testing is to evaluate and potentially confirm a diagnosis. For many diseases, early detection can facilitate improved treatment. Diagnostic tests vary, but they can often provide information in advance of the development of more severe disease, thereby allowing patients and their physicians to decide on courses of treatment. Likewise, a negative test may also provide some sense of relief and potentially be used to rule out alternative causes of symptoms. For SARS-CoV-2, the diagnostic value of testing was often limited. If one were to receive a positive PCR test, how would that change standards of care if there were limited (or no) treatment options available with demonstrated improvement in outcomes. The absence of evidence did not stop some people from pushing for miracle cures, such as hydroxychloroquine in 2020. This antimalarial drug is also used to treat lupus but was shown to be ineffective against severe outcomes of COVID-19 and to potentially pose cardiac risks to those who take it.[3,4] In 2021, others pushed to treat COVID-19 with ivermectin, a parasitic deworming agent intended for horses, despite it being shown to be ineffective and toxic in humans.[5,6] Efforts to push back against misinformation schemes to promote the equivalent of COVID-19 treatment snake oil were often met with fierce resistance whether through official governmental channels in 2020 or through a mix of organized and organic forms of online harassment. Notably, Rick Bright, the head of the Biomedical Advanced Research and Development Agency, was demoted from his position in April 2020.[7] His removal was reportedly linked to his resistance to Trump administration efforts to redirect even more funds to the use of hydroxychloroquine to treat those with test-confirmed COVID-19.

Even if testing could not be used as a precursor to prescribe a miracle cure, it could be used to assess impact: How many individuals were infected, how many were hospitalized, and finally, how many died of COVID-19? This type of testing measured the impact of suffering. And in doing so, it became a benchmark for failure. But former president Trump's remarks also reveal a far wider misconception regarding the difference between an infection and a case.[8] And they miss a deeper point, which is to use tests for an altogether different purpose. Tests can be used not just for diagnosis, and not just as a benchmark of failure, but as a means to reduce cases at the source.

At Scale: Testing As a Means of Mitigation

The reason for large-scale event restrictions, lockdowns, mask mandates, testing initiatives, and the rapid development of vaccines was simply because the threat of COVID-19 has never been about infections. The threat is that so many individuals who become infected become a confirmed COVID-19 case with clinician-detectable symptoms, and then, some of those become hospitalized, some are intubated, and some die. Yet, assessing impact based on fatalities alone is too narrow a measure. Ideally, accurately estimating current and prospective cases can help to forecast hospital load and scale-up public health interventions and preparedness appropriately—saving lives requires making sure hospitals can in fact handle and treat incoming caseloads.

So then, why test? First, the actual number of infections was not driven up by testing. Imagine a world in which it was not possible to conclusively identify the viral origin of unusual clusters of pneumonia-like illnesses, characterized by fever, cough, and eventually respiratory distress, as well as other symptoms include fatigue, myocarditis, and altered mental status. Even if we could not identify specific illnesses through molecular testing, individuals would still be sick, some would be hospitalized, and others would die (whether in or out of hospital settings). In that event, perhaps one would be forced to turn to other metrics, like in the Bills of Mortality recorded in seventeenth-century England, where prominent causes of death included "Feaver, Confumption, and Stopping of the Stomach."[9] In modern terms, even if a definitive diagnosis of COVID-19 was not possible, one could still measure its collective impact in terms of excess mortality over the course of the year.[10]

Before 2020, the United States experienced a steady rise of fatalities each year, from approximately 2.5 million fatalities in 2011 to 2.85 million fatalities in 2019. Approximately 400,000 additional fatalities per year is, in part, a reflection of a growing population. This means that there should be approximately 55,000 deaths in a given week in the United States, with slight increases expected around the New Year and slight decreases expected in the summer months. These levels can then be extrapolated to the expected number of deaths in 2020 and 2021. If previous trends held, there should have been somewhere between 2.9 million to 3 million fatalities in 2020 and 2021.

Figure 5.1 provides a stark perspective on COVID-19's impact. The United States experienced an estimated 3.38 million and 3.46 million fatalities in 2020 and 2021, respectively. The difference represents the excess mortality, approximately 460,000 and 490,000 excess deaths in 2020 and 2021, respectively. What was the cause of this stark change in mortality patterns? The answer is all too well known: COVID-19. There were ~825,000 documented COVID-19 fatalities in the United States between February 2020 and December 2021.[11] The concordance between these two estimates reveals yet another fact: not only has COVID-19 driven the significant increase in excess deaths in the United States, but a significant number of fatalities have likely been caused by COVID-19, even if they were not documented. Unfortunately, case fatality rates continued to remain elevated, such that there were ~950,000 documented COVID-19 fatalities in the United States by the end of February 2022 and ~1.1 million documented COVID-19 fatalities by the end of January 2023.

The reality is that if we had not tested, the situation would have been even worse. Testing for SARS-CoV-2 was never just about cases. The

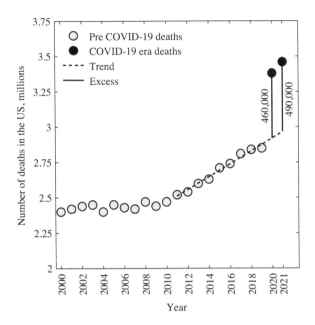

Figure 5.1. Estimate of excess deaths in the United States. Gray points denote data pre-COVID; solid black points denote data after pandemic emergence. The dashed line denotes a fit and extrapolation to 2020 and 2021, based on 2011–2019 data. The vertical lines illustrate the excess death estimates, 460,000 and 490,000 in 2020 and 2021, respectively. Alternative estimates of excess deaths depend on extrapolation to 2020 and 2021 in the absence of COVID-19 emergence. *Source*: CDC National Vital Statistics System. (2023). Excess deaths associated with COVID-19. https://www.cdc.gov/nchs/nvss/vsrr/covid19/excess_deaths.htm.

US public health establishment had a duty to understand (and confirm) what was making people sick. But testing had and has the ability to do far more. Testing can become part of an integrated approach to controlling spread and protecting vulnerable members of a community.

The Mitigation Potential of Pandemic Testing

Explaining why testing is part of the public health arsenal of defense requires revisiting how one case becomes many. Consider for a moment an asymptomatically infected individual. They have little to no idea they are infected. As a result, they are less likely to stay home, less likely to take preventative steps (like wearing a mask), and less likely to take precautions about whom they interact with. After exposure and infection, this asymptomatic individual will have a few days where they are infected but not infectious. A viral PCR test would likely turn up positive if that individual were to get tested. Likewise, an antigen test could be taken at home or at a clinic and inform individuals within minutes whether they are potentially infectious. Either way, the asymptomatic individual could be informed and choose to isolate themselves, dramatically reducing potential interactions that could lead to new infections. Even if the same individual were tested early during their infectious phase, then a majority of their potential for transmission would be reduced. Hence, more testing can actually lead to fewer cases if used as the basis for targeted action-taking.

Testing can also be used to help identify and mitigate potential chains of infection by focusing in on those most likely to have been exposed and potentially incubating a new infection. Individuals may learn of a friend, colleague, or family member with a confirmed case, usually because of symptoms that triggered a PCR or antigen test. Denote that person as the "primary case." If someone spent significant time indoors with a primary case without a mask, then the odds increase rapidly that the exposure led to a new transmission event. It typically takes a few days postinfection before a PCR test will reliably turn positive (the test delay is slightly longer for antigen tests). Hence, an individual may seek testing after being formally contacted by public health contact tracers or because they were personally informed by the person who likely infected them. In this idealized case, early testing could stop the chains of transmission from flowing ever farther outward (figure 5.2).

In this particular example, a single individual (the primary case) infects three others, yet those three are informed sufficiently early that they restrict contacts. The process is not perfect. One individual may have had interactions before isolation and ended up infecting one other person (the tertiary case). Nonetheless, rather than one case leading to three leading to nine, there would only be a single tertiary case linked to the primary case, and if testing is able to reach that tertiary case early enough, it is possible that this could mark the end of this particular

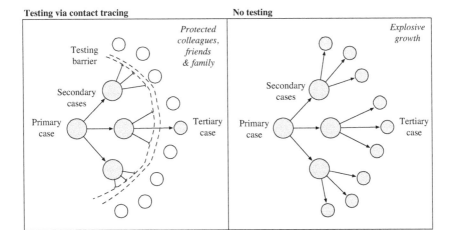

Figure 5.2. Schematic of the benefits of testing of close contacts (left) versus spread in the absence of testing (right). In the testing scenario, secondary cases are tested and isolated before spreading the virus to other individuals—in this example reducing spread to just one tertiary case. In the no-testing case, individuals may not know they are infected and infect others before symptoms lead to self-isolation—in this example leading to 9 tertiary cases.

transmission chain. Such an approach can work, in theory. In practice, there are barriers that span the availability of tests, the cost of testing, delays between testing and results, and the socioeconomic provisions for isolation.

For example, if not enough tests are available or cost money (and time to get) and—perhaps worse yet—if the results of the tests come back late, then the potential benefits rapidly diminish. The principles of why testing can work can be illustrated by focusing on any of the "secondary" cases in figure 5.2's left panel. Individuals who are infected progress through an exposed and then infectious stage. Imagine if a focal individual were tested on day 3 after infection, with a result returned on day 4, after which the individual was isolated. Even if they remained asymptomatic, then the potential transmission that could have taken place between days 4 and 14 could be reduced to nearly 0. Hence, if resources had been placed into large-scale deployment of testing, contact tracing, and support for paid time-off work and isolation, then perhaps this kind of focused testing could have worked to stop or slow exponential spread. This kind of strategy works if applied aggressively early—but not when the numbers of individuals to be contact-traced grows to outstrip public health capabilities.[12] But, of course, if the test is taken on day 3 and returned on day 10 (or 14), then the benefits of testing would have been lost. During the intervening period, the asymptomatic individual would already have moved about, interacted with others, and infected others. Unfortunately, such delays were far too often the case when using viral PCR tests. The key is that speed matters (figure 5.3).

The location, access, and cost of testing were far too great for much of 2020, and delays increased the perception that the utility of testing always came too late. In early to mid-2020, many testing sites came with a copay for the uninsured, and testing could cost upwards $75 per test.[13] (It is worth noting that the actual cost of testing is on the order of $5 to $10 per PCR sample and can be reduced even further at scale.[14]) In effect, even if the secondary cases in the preceding figure know that they are likely infected, the test results often come too late or were too costly in the first place to make a difference. Moreover, in many cases, individuals were infected in public settings or at events where contact tracing remained woefully incomplete. It can be difficult for many reasons, even with well-intentioned participants, to track down one's contacts. But, for many, the contact tracer's effort was

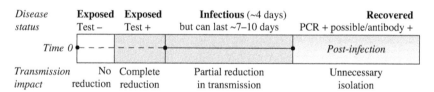

Figure 5.3. Schematic of the relationship between disease status and transmission impact. Individuals are considered to have one of three disease statuses: (i) exposed, (ii) infectious, or (iii) recovered. Exposed individuals are not infectious but can test positive for the disease either with a PCR test (at first) and then antigen tests (subsequently). Infectious individuals can transmit the virus and will test positive. Recovered individuals can no longer transmit but can test positive and will also almost certainly have antibodies that can be detected using serological tests. In essence, the timing of disease testing can have different effects on transmission.

yct another intrusion into their private lives and privacy. The delays in testing had their origins in mistakes made early on—including with the release of what had been intended to be the national standard for molecular viral tests: a PCR test kit designed and distributed by the Centers for Disease Control and Prevention (CDC).

The rapid spread of cases in China in December 2019 and January 2020 provided some notion of an early warning. If the United States could move fast enough, perhaps we could be better prepared to ward off the inevitable arrival of COVID-19 through international air travel.[15,16] To help test for SARS-CoV-2 at scale required some way to identify and screen individuals for the disease. This job—to design and deploy the template for a national testing strategy—fell to the CDC headquartered in Atlanta, Georgia. Unfortunately, this testing effort was flawed from the start. One of the key errors was not one of strategy but of practice: namely, the design and distribution of PCR testing kits by the CDC.[17]

As explained earlier, PCR testing uses molecular templates that are highly specific to a single type of target virus genetic material. If the RNA of the target virus taken from a sample is mixed in with the test kit, then a small segment of the genetic material of the virus will be replicated again and again, until it can be detected as a fluorescent signal in the laboratory and reported as a positive test result. It is vital that the test kits be accurate in two senses. First, the test should not inadvertently report a positive test signal when the specific viral genetic material is not present in the sample. Second, the test should report a positive test signal when the specific viral genetic material is present in the sample. Unfortunately, the CDC test kits had both a design and a production flaw. It has been hypothesized that the design flaw arose because the CDC division responsible for assay development used multiple target components of the genetic sequence that makes up the spike protein.[18] As it turned out, some of these sequences had very little cross-reactivity with the target viral RNA and instead reacted to other viral RNA. This means that a positive test using the diagnostic panel test developed by the CDC could not be safely interpreted as a true positive. The increase in false positives may have also been compounded by manufacturing errors and the fact that the CDC initially prevented others from developing their own tests.[19,20] In summary, the public was aware that the CDC's test kits were flawed soon after they distributed in early February 2020.[21] This lack of trust led to delays in the use of testing as a form of early warning and did something much worse: it undermined public trust in the CDC and in the concept of testing as part of a reliable, public health arsenal. As a result, instead of scaling up manufacturing of a nationally accepted standard, state health agencies, pharmaceutical companies, and universities had to develop alternatives that could be reliably used as a diagnostic assay. Developing such alternatives took time that could have been used for impactful mitigation.

As illustrated in figure 5.2, an accurate, diagnostic assay can play a role in mitigation only if results are returned quickly. Here again, the United States failed to follow through on basic epidemiological principles. If a test takes 1 day to return positive or negative results, then that is 1 day out of a potentially 7- to 10-day period of future infection. In this way, the majority of potential infection can be avoided through the rapid return of test results followed by isolation. Roughly speaking if an individual is likely to infect 3 others, the cumulative impacts of mitigation must be reduced by a factor of 2/3 or more so that cases tend to decrease on average, rather than increase. In this way, rather than infecting 3 individuals on average, a primary case might only infect 1 (or 0)—leading to less than one new case on average and the decline of cases overall. But, if test results were delayed, then action-taking would also be delayed, and the narrow window to make a difference would be lost. As a result, if testing was to make a difference, speed matters.[22]

For example, assuming that transmission was distributed randomly across the entire ~10-day infectious period, then contact tracing, testing, return of results, and isolation would have to be fast, ideally ~3–5 days after the infection to catch individuals in the earlier part of their infectious period (see figure 5.3). This kind of reactive testing is ambitious, and it is also prone to supply chain delays, logistic challenges, and the varied willingness of individuals to participate (and of contact tracers to reconstruct contacts). In practice, the United States failed to execute and deliver rapid turnaround of results.[23] Surveys taken in mid-2020 reported that only 25% those who had PCR tests received results on the same or next day, with nearly 40% receiving them after 4 or more days (figure 5.4). These delays represent a lower bound on the actual delays between infection and the return of results. Because of delays to get testing, the cumulative effect of delays means that tests no longer became a meaningful form of mitigation at the population scale. Moreover, in some cases, delays became so long that they no longer even provide guidance with a diagnosis given the time during which symptoms appear.

Recognizing the potential for testing to make a difference as a form of mitigation, a number of companies tried to develop contact-tracing apps to try and accelerate the time between exposure, contact, and

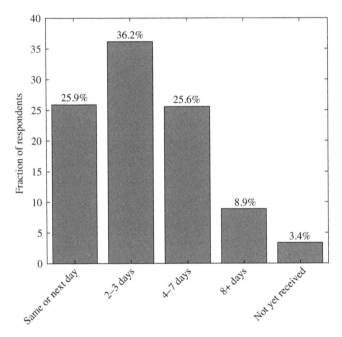

Figure 5.4. Survey responses to the delay between testing and receipt of results, in summer 2020 in the United States. Survey was conducted through a collaboration between CNBC and Dynata. *Source*: Tirrell, M., Wells, N., and Miller, L. (2020, August 15). Forty percent of US Covid-19 tests come back too late to be clinically meaningful, data show. CNBC. https://www.cnbc.com/2020/08/15/forty-percent-of-us -covid-19-tests-come-back-too-late-to-be-clinically-meaningful-data-show.html.

testing. Here again, the United States failed. A national-level app was never developed. Instead, individual states (and some companies) launched competing platforms. Yet, such apps require a critical threshold of individuals to participate for them to work effectively. For example, these apps commonly use Bluetooth signals between phones as a distance detector. In effect, the communication between phones passively collects information proximity. So, if one individual were to be infected and add information to the contact-tracing app, then other individuals who spent an extended amount of time with the infected individual would automatically receive a notification of exposure (without informing them of the identity of the infected individual). But such exposure systems require large-scale participation. If you are one of a few people to sign up, then the probability decreases that a contact is notified or that you are notified of exposures among your nonparticipating contacts—the digital contact-tracing system fails to notify the people it should. There are also real challenges with privacy; private information on one's health is being broadcast to proximity-based contacts, and information on proximity could also potentially be misused. In practice, the United States never implemented a national, digital contact-tracing initiative to connect to testing—unlike the United Kingdom.[24] As a result, even if rapid contact tracing could lead to interventional testing of contacts, the magnitude of testing was far too low. There were approximately 250 million viral tests performed in the United States in 2020 alone.[25] As big as that number sounds, that is still less than one test per person in the entire year!

Yet thinking in terms of population scales points to a radically different way to approach testing. This new approach goes beyond confirmation of a symptom-based diagnosis and the initiation of contact tracing. Instead, the idea is to use testing irrespective of symptoms in order to control outbreaks. The principle of such efforts runs completely counter to claims that more testing means more cases. Instead, if implemented effectively, more testing can actually mean many *fewer* cases. If entire groups of individuals are tested regularly, it is possible to reduce the effective number of potential new infections and control local chains of transmission. With sufficient resources, it may even be possible to control population-level outbreaks to levels below that using conventional mitigation approaches or contact tracing.

Scaling Up Pandemic Testing

The utility of testing to slow epidemic spread comes down to a question of scale and consequences. For the individuals being tested, the test result is the same whether or not they are one of a few or one of many being tested. But, collectively, many tests can have a nonlinear and, indeed, outsized impact on the spread of the epidemic as a whole.

The rationale begins with the basic modalities of transmission. Part 1 of this book laid out how asymptomatic transmission could lead paradoxically to worse overall outcomes at the population scale. At one extreme, if nearly everyone was asymptomatic, then even though many get infected, very few have symptomatic infections, and even fewer become severely ill or die. If nearly every infection leads to a symptomatic infection (and transmission is linked to symptoms), then recognition of symptoms and post-symptom isolation can reduce the chance of spread. This means that those unlucky enough to be infected can have bad outcomes—including severe cases, hospitalizations, or fatalities—but the disease does not spread to as many people. The severity at the population level requires multiplying two factors together: the number of people infected and the chance of a severe outcome if infected. At one extreme—the asymptomatic limit—the severe outcome is reduced. At the other extreme—the symptomatic limit—the number of infections is reduced. It is in the middle where the two factors multiplied together lead to the worse overall outcome. Yet this is where there is an opportunity for testing to make a difference.

Testing interrupts the period over which individuals can transmit their infection to others, if it is used as a basis for isolation and/or contact reduction. Testing frequently enough means that there is a chance to catch an infection in the presymptomatic stage or even among individuals who have sufficiently mild/asymptomatic cases that they will never develop recognizable symptoms but will nonetheless infect others. But how much testing is enough? And are such testing levels feasible? Let us examine the answers to these questions one by one.

First, we can estimate the approximate impact of testing at the population scale by asking, What is the chance that someone will be tested before their infectious period concludes? The chance depend on several factors: (i) the typical period of being exposed, (ii) the typical period of infectiousness, (iii) the frequency of testing (and return of results), and (iv) the sensitivity of testing. If we examine each of these factors, we have a chance to understand the scale necessary to affect outbreak size at the population level (i.e., using testing as a part of mitigation). In doing so, it is important to separate out different kinds of tests because their use depends on particular features of what they measure. But, to start, let us focus again on what is considered the gold standard for testing: PCR-based viral testing.

A PCR test indicates whether or not an individual is shedding viral RNA. This requires that the individual has sufficient viral genome copies inside them that it can be detected by a test: a process that usually takes a single turnaround day for saliva or nasal-swab samples. There may even be a window of a few days where an individual would test positive but would unlikely be infectious. Assume that early detection period lasts 2 days. Now, imagine that individuals are tested at random, irrespective of their symptom status with a frequency of once every 10 days. Then there is approximately a 2/10 (or 20%) chance that they will be tested in this period. Although the probabilities are small, if caught early enough, such testing would eliminate all or nearly all of the expected transmission from such individuals. But, for this to happen, the test must be sensitive enough and the test results must be returned fast enough.

The choice of the word *sensitive* rather than a catchall term like accuracy is intentional. The sensitivity of a test denotes the probability that an individual who truly has the condition (in this case, infected with SARS-CoV-2) will return a positive test result. Likewise, the word *specificity* denotes the probability that a test will return a negative result if the person does not have the condition. Ideally, both the sensitivity and specificity would be 1 (or in equivalent terms 100%), but such ideal cases do not apply in the real world. If a PCR test has 99% sensitivity, this means that the test would return a positive result 99/100 times, in the event that the individual actually is infected. In reality, test sensitivity varies depending on the time since infection. Initially, after infection, PCR test sensitivity is nearly 0 and then rises to above 99% during the infectious period. This level of sensitivity stands in contrast to antigen tests, which require the binding of viral proteins in a sample to antibodies on a rapid diagnostic kit. Such tests may have lower sensitivities during the infectious period and a longer period where they return false negative results.[26] But antigen tests do have a marked advantage: speed.

Consequently, for testing to make an impact at the population scale, we can return to the individual scale and see the extent to which potential transmission is reduced. There is a tension here between the time it takes to identify an infected case with testing and the amount of future transmission that can be prevented with a diagnostic test. Figure 5.5 highlights this point graphically.

The tension is a balance of two effects. On the one hand, because of increasing test sensitivity over time, a test taken too early may yield a negative result. In contrast, a viral test taken a few days after infection

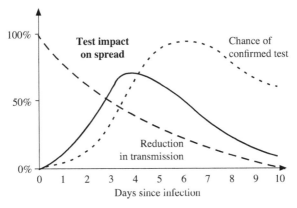

Figure 5.5. Schematic of test impact on individual spread as a function of days since infection. The individual-level impact is a product of the chance of a confirmed test (dotted curve) multiplied by the reduction in transmission when a positive test is followed by isolation (dashed curve). Impact peaks a few days after infection.

is more likely to yield a positive and remain positive up to 10 days after the initial exposure. An antigen test is likely to turn positive later and then turn negative earlier—more closely corresponding to the infectious period. The other tension is that the impact of testing goes down with time since exposure. If it were possible to identify an infection in the first day after exposure, likely during the preinfectious period, then all forward transmission would be reduced. Yet, if one catches a case at the end of the infectious period, then hardly any (or perhaps none at all) of the forward transmission is reduced. These two tensions are shown in the dotted and dashed curves, respectively, in figure 5.5. Their combination suggests that most of the population-level benefits will accrue for those tests taken a few days after infection.

But how does one know one's infection time? In practice, this is hard to do, given the significant levels of asymptomatic transmission. In effect, many (if not most) people have no idea when they were exposed no who infected them. As a result, they cannot necessarily time their testing to coincide with a few days after exposure. Precisely for this reason, a number of universities began to consider a different approach—large-scale asymptomatic testing.[27,28,29] These efforts were managed and developed largely independently, although the developers of these testing approaches were often in contact behind the scenes to share methodologies, preliminary findings, and strategies to put these ideas into practice.[30]

The idea is to aggressively use tests at a much larger scale to try and reduce transmission, rather than wait to selectively use tests in the event that someone suspects they have been exposed or are showing symptoms (and therefore seeking testing). The epidemiological principle is that testing will sometimes coincide with moments before or after the infectious period, but if used frequently enough, testing will be more likely to coincide with the preinfectious or early infectious period. Notably, if the period of testing is on the order of a week, then it is almost certain that an individual who happens to be exposed will test positive, even if they are asymptomatic and have no awareness that they are infected. If the test happens to be in the early stages of infection, then the number of secondary cases for that isolated individual may be reduced to nearly 0. Whereas, if the test happens to be in the later stages of infection, then the number of secondary cases is only slightly reduced. Overall, individuals may be tested in fixed or random-ized schedules, given testing capacity, with the net effect being that there is a chance to reduce outbreak size if implementing testing at scale. Figure 5.6 illustrates the principle schematically.

Here, a population of students is considered to be in distinct compartments—similar to the core epidemiological modeling idea in-troduced in chapter 3. The use of testing brings with it a new category: those who test positive and are isolated. We assume in our example that the test is of sufficiently high specificity that only infectious individu-als test positive and are placed in isolation: thoughtful approaches to test specificity, sensitivity, and speed of test results constitute a key part of real-world implementation.[31] The new compartment Q is where test-ing makes a difference. Those students who test positive and are iso-lated (whether because they are symptomatic or asymptomatic) are at significantly lower risk of infecting others. This reduces the number of cases per infection and the population-averaged effective reproduc-tion number.

This model has a key new parameter: the rate of testing (including the return of test results) relative to the infectious period. If testing occurs at a timescale on the order of (or faster than) the infectious pe-riod, then testing can make a significant impact. That is, given a 10-day infectious period, testing on the order of once a week (or in some

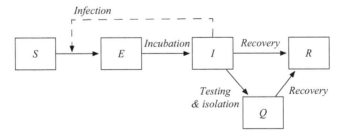

Figure 5.6. Compartments of susceptible (S), exposed (E), infectious (I), quaran-tined/isolated (Q), and recovered (R) individuals in a population, where testing competes with the natural recovery period to move individuals into an isolation category, thereby reducing the chance of new infections.

circumstances, twice a week) can significantly reduce the chance for spread, whereas testing every other week or month or once per academic term will have little to no impact on controlling spread (even if it provides some peace of mind). The core idea is straightforward: testing frequently, irrespective of symptoms, can actually reduce new cases—but to do so requires a system for large-scale testing and an environment to evaluate the potential for the use of testing as a form of mitigation.

Testing in Practice at US College Campuses

In the late spring and summer of 2020, a number of university campuses across the United States decided to embark on a rapid response effort: to develop the internal capacity to test for COVID-19 at scale. The rationale was that they would be able to identify enough cases early enough to reduce R_0 from 3 to less than 1 (on average), enabling a safer return to dense, live-learn environments. The rationale combined the simple principle of test-based interception of cases and population-based model projections. These projection and associated models have to make a number of simplifying assumptions, and the resulting models varied in complexity. Nonetheless, they all shared a common principle: a combination of fast results and high sensitivity was the key to ensuring that tests could identify an infected individual well before that individual recovered and, in some cases, before that person was even infectious.

Figure 5.7 represents one such modeling study. It is based on work that I shared with colleagues and the leadership at Georgia Tech in the summer of 2020 to explain why testing at scale could help protect our community, in light of the expected return of students to campus in August 2020.[32]

This contour plot is the result of simulating an epidemiological model in a college campus while testing at different rates (as denoted on the y-axis) and assuming that entry testing was used to reduce cases at the start of the semester. More detailed models, including individual behavior were incorporated into other university responses

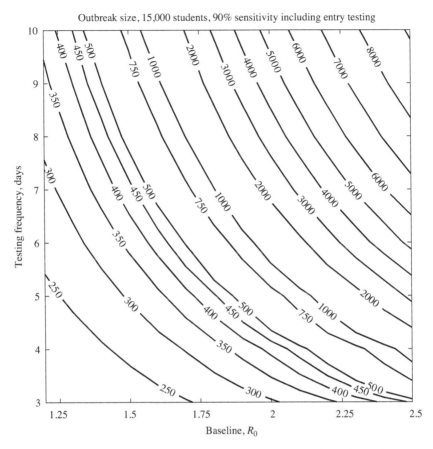

Outbreak size, 15,000 students, 90% sensitivity including entry testing

Figure 5.7. Epidemic modeling of the predicted cumulative number of cases in one 14-week semester expected to occur on campus. A simplified SEIR (susceptible-exposed-infected-removed) model assumed a total community of 15,000 individuals, a two-day latent period on average between infection and positivity, and a two-day average infectious period. Transmission rates were varied to yield the basic reproduction number (R_0) on the x-axis, including entry testing and a 90% sensitive test. Contour lines show the expected number of cases given covariation in average test frequency per individual and the baseline transmission ratio. We shared the data with campus leadership to argue for the implementation of a testing program and with the community in our communication efforts in August 2020.

(e.g., at the University of Illinois at Urbana-Champaign).[33] The contour lines denote the total number of infections in a campus community of 15,000 given changes in the basic reproduction number (x-axis) and the testing frequency (in days). The basic reproduction number is hypothesized to be smaller than at the start of the outbreak, in part because of measures taken to prevent transmission in gatherings—including a large-scale effort by faculty, staff, and students to advocate for requiring masks in classrooms and shared spaces.[34] For every combination of values, an epidemic model can be simulated that incorporates reduce transmission for those who have tested positive.

As is apparent, more frequent testing reduces the expected size of outbreaks from many thousands to approximately hundreds or ~1,000 in a campus of approximately 15,000 students and staff. Notably, testing can be synergistic with other mitigation measures. The contours depict the expected number of cases with different levels of mitigation, as shown on the x-axis. The idea is that individuals are likely to infect fewer individuals if mask-wearing, social distancing, and online courses are also in place. These strategic intervention measures are synergistic with testing. In practice, the Georgia Tech system worked. It worked because a large community came together on short notice to translate theoretical ideas into reality, often overcoming significant technical and logistical challenges. The same process happened at dozens of institutions nationwide. In practice, the University of Illinois at Urbana-Champaign (UIUC), the University of California San Diego (UCSD), Georgia Tech, Duke, Yale, Harvard, the Air Force Academy, the University of Washington, and many other universities initiated their own asymptomatic-based testing and intervention programs. In each case, students, staff, and faculty joined together to build up capacity when neither the federal government nor private industry was able to meet the demand. Explaining this logistical challenge helps to shed light on what went right and what went wrong, and it allows us to reconsider the use of testing moving forward.

The US research institutions form a national, geographically distributed network of world-class scientific research hubs. The leading "R1" universities typically have elite biomedical facilities and are often associated with medical and public health schools that have built-in capacity for diagnostic testing as part of their campus-associated hospital.[35] Even those without an affiliated medical school have many labs that use PCR methods as a bread-and-butter type of diagnostic test in their non-COVID research activities. As a result, developing a reliable PCR-based assay to test for the presence of SARS-CoV-2 was not rocket science, at least not for many dozens of research universities and associated biological research institutions. The assay development used either saliva (as at UIUC, Georgia Tech, Emory, Penn, Princeton, and Yale) or nasal-swabs (as at UCSD and Duke) as the basis for testing the entire community. The premise in all of these tests is that students self-provide a sample using a test kit, including a buffer that immediately deactivates viruses (if they are present) but allows for the preservation of viral genetic material that is the target of the PCR test. Then, these tests are aggregated or "pooled" to reduce costs and improve speed of preliminary results (given low incidence),[36] brought to a laboratory and tested initially, with results typically returned the following day (or, in some cases, the same day). Although universities differed in approach, the consensus typically was to aim to have all students tested at least once a week; to isolate students, staff, and faculty who tested positive; and then to leverage the test information to initiate contact tracing.

The question becomes, then: How does one interpret the results from individual tests? If the goal of testing is to control spread, then it is likely that testing platforms are being deployed in a university campus community where the actual prevalence of the disease can be quite low. This presents some unique challenges. First, it is important to use tests with very high specificities. Recall that the specificity denotes the probability that someone who does not have COVID-19 tests negative. Hence, a 99.5% specific test implies that 1 in 200 tests would turn up positive, even if no one had the disease, whereas a 99% specific test implies that 1 in 100 tests would turn up positive, even if no one had the disease. Finally, if a PCR test had a 99.9% specificity, then only 1 in 1,000 tests would turn up positive, even if no one had the disease. But, in populations where most people will not have the disease, even those small probabilities can have an impact on what is termed the "positive predictive value."

Consider a case where the actual prevalence of the disease was approximately 0.5% (or 1 in 200 people are infected), and the test has a

99% sensitivity and a 99.5% specificity. In this case, then surprisingly (and counterintuitively), one would expect approximately 10 positive tests for every 1,000 individuals tested. Of these 10 positive tests, 5 would be true positives and 5 would be false positives. How can this be? If 1 in 200 is actually infected, we expect 5 to be actually infected in a group of 1,000—and given the high sensitivity, we can reasonably assume that each of those 5 individuals receive a positive test result. But because of the 99.5% specificity, then 1 in 200 individuals who are actually negative end up testing positive. This leads to 5 more positive tests, albeit from individuals who are not infected. But we do not know who is who. In effect, if you had a positive result, there would only be a 50% chance you were actually infected! This is not how most people (or medical doctors) think about diagnostic tests—especially tests that have putatively high accuracies! And this is also one of the reasons that early serological surveys of the kind described in chapter 1 were so fraught with the potential for confusion.[37]

As a result, most institutions ended up adopting a two-stage approach. First, samples could be divided up and pooled together in different combinations both to reduce the number of PCR tests used but also to provide a double confirmation of an initial test positive. Pooling mixes samples together in different combinations. Pools are comprised of unique sets of samples, so if pool A and pool B both come back positive, it is likely that there is a singular cause: a particular individual sample that was placed into both the A and B pools. At this point, it is possible to inform an individual that their surveillance test has been referred to diagnostic testing. This strategy also reduces the number of times that samples have to be subject to a full "CLIA" testing protocol. CLIA stands for Clinical Laboratory Improvement Amendments, and it represents a standard of quality and lab controls evaluated by the Centers for Medicare and Medicaid Services in order to perform diagnostic tests on human samples.[38] Many universities have CLIA labs in place, while others (like Georgia Tech) had to build up capacity and pass certification review quickly, even as the demand for testing ramped up in advance of students returning for the new semester. By using pooled samples, one can reduce costs, return advisory (albeit not medically approved) results faster, and then conduct follow-up CLIA-approved tests on those samples identified in the original pools. CLIA-approved test positives could then be shared with the individual who tested as well as reported to cognizant state public health agencies, triggering the initiation of contact tracing as well as other mitigation approaches meant to slow down spread.

In effect, a number of US research institutions ended up building their own capacity to test a campus community on a weekly basis (if not faster). Although certain Ivy League universities and even some public universities were able to mandate testing requirements, the case of Georgia Tech is particularly instructive because the testing was not mandated due to the University System of Georgia's centralized approach to governance. More broadly, mandates on masks, testing, and vaccines remain controversial in the United States—an issue to be returned to later in this chapter and in chapter 6. Nonetheless, even without a mandate, many people participated, and the participation made a difference. First, the majority of positive cases identified at Georgia Tech were found through the asymptomatic testing system rather than through symptomatic-based testing (62% of all cases were identified through asymptomatic surveillance testing). Second, the actual outbreaks on campus were identified early and short-circuited, meaning that Georgia Tech experienced far fewer cases than expected—in line with the modeling-based justifications for the program.[39]

One comparative illustration of impact is to contrast Georgia Tech's system with that of the nearby University of Georgia in Athens (UGA), the state's flagship land grant university. The two universities had vastly different test capacities, despite being just 90 minutes away from each other. Georgia Tech averaged ~10,000 tests per week in fall 2020, whereas UGA with approximately twice the number of students averaged half as many tests. At Georgia Tech, the positivity rate rose to approximately 4% in early September 2020 and then rapidly declined to less than 1%, where it remained for nearly the entire fall 2020 term. In contrast, positivity rates approached nearly 9% at UGA and remained above 4% for weeks afterward. Positivity rate denotes the fraction of tests in the population that return a positive result. If everyone in a population were tested, the positivity rate would be a good estimate of the overall prevalence of the disease (i.e., the fraction of people who are infected). But not everyone gets tested. When tests are scarce or not encouraged for asymptomatic individuals, then people tend to get tested when they suspect they may be infected. Hence, the positivity rate is almost invariably higher than the actual prevalence—especially when tests are limited. But, for asymptomatic testing schemes, positivity levels are more reflective of what could be considered a population survey of how many people are infected at any given moment. Having nearly 10% of a community infected at a given time is enormously high (and should not be compared to positivity rates on the test-limited and symptomatic-based approaches taken by states). By testing more, Georgia Tech identified cases earlier and was able to isolate individuals, which helped to reduce transmission until vaccines were widely available to young adults in spring 2021 (figure 5.8).

That is good news. But it comes with an enormous caveat. When viral testing was scarce elsewhere, university students, staff, and faculty at Georgia Tech could get a saliva-based test weekly for free, often with a snack as an inducement, and have results returned to them in a day.[40] This was not the case at UGA—where tests were less frequent and not at the scale necessary to represent effective mitigation. Moreover, the University System of Georgie has 26 member institutions, and the testing programs at the other universities were either scarce or nonexistent. Two years into the pandemic, there were approximately 16 million PCR-based molecular viral tests conducted in the state of Georgia (population: 10.6 million) and approximately 500,000 PCR-based molecular viral tests conducted at Georgia Tech (community size: 30,000). Per capita, that amounts to 1.5 tests per person every two years in the state and 15 tests per person every two years at the technical university located in the state's capitol. This 10-fold difference represents an enormous opportunity, provided testing can become part of our collective pandemic prevention strategy rather than a feature of specialized universities and a barometer for collective failure.

The more we test, the more infections we find. Rather than an admonition against testing, this truism can lead to action-taking, particularly if we are willing to extend this pithy statement into one infused with actual meaning for public health. Here, instead, is an alternative:

> The more we test, the more infections we find in the short term, which can lead to fewer severe cases in the long term.

Testing for testing's sake does little good. Indeed, it can even do harm. For example, finding out one is positive for COVID-19 without the benefits of health care, paid leave, or contact tracing simply means that individuals are left on their own to deal with a diagnosis. If they suffer economic losses when they are forced to stay home by public health policies that are not reinforced by economic policies, it will make them less likely to test in the future. Instead, when testing is combined with realistic action-taking, then we are more likely to engage individuals, increase their willingness to test, and reduce the chance that an individual who has an asymptomatic/mild case ends up infecting many others. To get there, we need to use a variety of tests and responses rather than expecting a single test modality to act as a silver bullet and halt the pandemic on its own. Each test comes with limitations. Layering imperfect tests together can achieve in aggregate what one test cannot do alone. In the next section, we explore multiple test modalities that could be used in combination to achieve different aims—from understanding the epidemic state to controlling spread in vulnerable communities and ultimately facilitating safer interactions as part of a better normal.

Action Opportunity: Doing More Testing, Preventing More Cases

Action-taking requires information—information that will increasingly become harder to obtain in the absence of support for public health infrastructure and data-sharing agreements that tell us who is infected, where, and at what levels. The foundations are in place to establish a

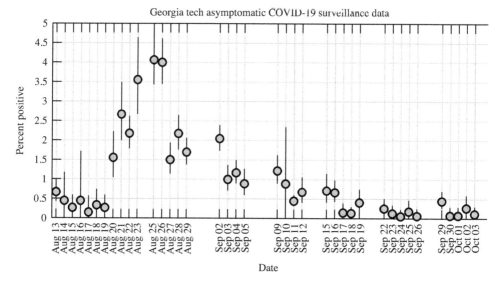

Figure 5.8. Surveillance positive rate increased from ~0.5% to 4% and then decreased to <1% except for a brief period post-Halloween 2020. *Source*: Data from Georgia Tech COVID-19 dashboard, archived at https://health.gatech.edu/archived-monitoring -covid-19-dashboard/, following methods described in Gibson, G. et al. (2022) Surveillance-to-diagnostic testing program for asymptomatic SARS-CoV-2 infections on a large, urban campus in Fall 2020. *Epidemiology* 33: 209–216. https://doi.org/10 .1097/EDE.0000000000001448

sustainable testing infrastructure building on two primary modalities that have been scaled up in response to COVID-19 and that have helped us understand "community spread." Of course, community spread may be in the eye of the beholder. Formally speaking, the CDC adopted a holistic metric of community spread that combines two key measurements: (i) how many new cases have been reported in the past week and (ii) the intensity of recent COVID-19 related hospital admissions and bed use.[41] This metric was later expanded to include (iii) the community-wide vaccination coverage.[42] Community spread metrics integrate both case number and likely severity. In practice, this metric depends on test reports. As a result, if the pipeline of testing dries up, then we will lose the ability to take steps to inform communities as a whole and, potentially, diminish our ability to protect hospital resources. Optimistically, breaking down community spread

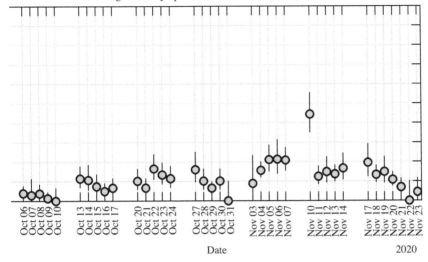

Georgia tech asymptomatic COVID-19 surveillance data

Date   2020

Figure 5.8. continued

into cases and severe outcomes also provides a mechanism to explore how to prioritize resources and how to do more with less.

Beginning in summer 2020, multiple universities in the United States instituted campus-wide testing programs. These programs became a benchmark for using large-scale asymptomatic testing to understand the overall state of the epidemic and then to systematically intervene—for example, using tests as a means to trigger case isolation, quarantine, and changes in the delivery of courses. From the perspective of an intervention, more is indeed better (at least within a certain limit). More testing increases the chances that individuals can be identified to be infected in the asymptomatic or presymptomatic phases and isolated from the community. This test-and-isolate procedure reduces the chances that an infected individual can infect others. These intensive systems, often built on a PCR-based accurate viral testing platform, were able in many cases to hold prevalence to less than 1% at any given moment even amid intensive community spread.

If our goal is understanding the epidemic state in order to inform decision-makers and the public on how to take action, then it is possible to do nearly as well with far fewer tests—especially if the sampling of tests are done in a thoughtful way. Let us envision a scenario where 1 in 200 individuals is infected (a prevalence of 0.5%). In that case, a city of 200,000 (about the size of Richmond, Virginia, or Spokane, Washington) would have approximately 1,000 individuals infected at a given moment in time. Testing every individual in the population weekly using a high-quality PCR test would cost $2 million a week if done at scale and with internal platforms (assuming a cost of $10/test) or closer to $10 million a week if using a commercial platform (assuming $50/test). By comparison, the annual operating budget of Spokane[43] and Richmond[44] range between $800 million to $1 billion a year. Hence, an annual testing program would cost at least $100 million a year—and it would almost certainly lead to problems. The same holds true even if adopting antigen testing at scale. Testing a population with a prevalence of 0.5% would require the use of highly specific tests. For example, a test with 99.5% specificity would generate approximate 1,000 true positives and 1,000 false positives when testing a population the size of Richmond or Spokane. Hence, 50% of positive test results would in fact not be infected—leading to a false positive rate of 50%, despite the use of a highly accurate test—for the same reasons as explained in the earlier section. Even if a highly specific test (on the order of 99.9% specific) were used, then there would still be on the order of 1,000 true positives and 200 false positives—a false positive rate of 200/1200, equivalent to 1 in 6. The logistics, sustainability, costs, and practical implications of a large-scale asymptomatic testing program in a relatively low prevalence population argue against its use as a mean to estimate the epidemic state for the population at large. But there is another way—by using a combination of voluntary testing, rapid testing, testing surveys, and environmental-based testing (including wastewater surveillance) to assess case prevalence. The aim is to use the data we have to estimate the information we want; that is, how many people are infected and how such infections are heterogeneously distributed across location, age, gender, race/ethnicity, and socioeconomic status.

Thus far, the number of reported cases has been used as a proxy for the actual intensity of community spread. The number of reported cases represents a significant underestimate of infections, however, given asymptomatic infections and the logistical challenges in testing. Hence, crudely, one way to estimate prevalence is to use gaps between cases and fatalities along with documented infection fatality rate (IFR) values to infer the prevalence—a process that becomes harder with time as IFR shifts in vaccinated communities. Another way to estimate prevalence is to use the gap between the cumulative number of documented cases and the number of individuals with antibodies to recalibrate and turn documented cases into an estimate of actual cases.[45] But, over time, relying on this type of constant scaling factor will almost certainly prove problematic. What happens if individuals tune out and stop testing, or if testing capacity degrades—whether through neglect, passively, or actively? Alternatively, what happens if individuals test at home and those tests are no longer reported to public health authorities?[46] Long-term efforts to prevent future pandemics require an infrastructure solution.

Another way to estimate the number of individuals infected would be to take a polling approach. In conventional polling, a large enough and representative enough group is identified, their "status" is evaluated (for polls, that will be a political preference, and for prevalence, that would be their infection status), and then the results are scaled up to the population at large by trying to correct biases inherent in the representation of the sample. Political polls can have errors, sometimes beyond those expected, but they are also more error-prone because of the winner-takes-all nature of most US elections. In the case of an infection survey, the point is not to say whether more than 50% of the population is infected but to estimate the fraction. As a result, surveys on the orders of hundreds (or perhaps thousands) could be used—with care taken to distribute and engage (potentially marginalized) communities that are unlikely to seek out voluntary testing. In this way, the estimating problem could become an expense costing a few thousand dollars a week for the test apparatus, run by a dedicated program manager connecting with local (potentially university) laboratories, with material and labor costs of a few hundred thousand dollars a year rather than a few hundred million dollars a year. Such an investment could have many other ancillary benefits, including engaging more individuals in health surveys, extending community health care, and providing the infrastructure to address the emergence of localized pandemics. Such efforts have been implemented in the United Kingdom.[47] Over time, thoughtful use of testing data could also allow local officials to modulate the intensity of sampling based on previous surveys—decreasing intensity in periods of low spread and increasing them in periods of higher spread when careful attention is needed to protect vulnerable communities. Such an investment could also help ground-truth and calibrate a scalable option: wastewater surveillance testing.

What goes in, must come out. The adage applies to pathogens as well as food or many drugs. The collective signatures of our pathogen loads can be found in wastewater. Wastewater testing takes samples from sewer lines, filters them, and then takes filtered samples and applies the same principles used to detect SARS-CoV-2 in an individual patient sample—namely, using molecular templates to try and find a viral needle in a haystack. Unfortunately, considering how many people have had COVID, finding the viral signal has been easy, to the point that signals of community spread in wastewater often mirror the signal derived from test results.[48] What does this mean? In practice, linking wastewater testing with community testing could lead to a calibration curve. A calibration curve would allow public health officials to translate the signal of SARS-CoV-2 RNA measured in wastewater to the equivalent number of active infections in a focal area.[49] The principle of such calibration is the same when thinking about other types of sensors. Full community viral sampling is challenging and often leads to biased outcomes. In contrast, measuring SARS-CoV-2 RNA and other pathogen signatures in wastewater is relatively easy from a technical perspective—though extending such approaches in (rural) communities disconnected from sewer lines presents challenges.

If developed, calibration curves that link viral RNA to cases could allow for point-of-time sampling at select points in a sanitation network as a means to estimate the number (and even location) of infected individuals in a focal community.[50] This approach requires national standards, local implementation, and cooperation between local, state, and national health authorities to enable responsive interpretation of wastewater signals. There is an enormous potential in wastewater surveillance precisely because it integrates across people and pathogens. Moreover, such wastewater systems can also have ancillary benefits, potentially for detecting the emergence and change in viral variants, including cryptic lineages.[51] Of course, understanding the state of play of the pandemic is one thing—knowing how to intervene in high-impact settings is another. Testing can play a role there, too.

Action Opportunity: Controlling Risk in Vulnerable Communities

COVID-19 has been a strange disease. Many have been infected unwittingly, never knowing (or at least never confirming) that they were infected.[52] Others ended up with challenging cases that eventually resolve over the course of a week, whereas others remain affected by debilitating symptoms that remain both underexplored and underexplained and in need of intensive follow-up study.[53] But through it all, one feature has remained salient: many millions of people worldwide have died from a disease that is approximately 100-fold less lethal than Ebola—at least when judged at the individual scale.

In total, approximately 1 in 300 Americans died in a little over two years because of a disease that just as often leads to a mild or asymptomatic case as it leads to a symptomatic or severe case. But as already described in part 1, the severity is not distributed equally. Although many factors influence the course of an infection, one factor stands out: age. As was already described, these age-dependent impacts become intensified when many older (and often medically frail) individuals live together and are then accidentally exposed to the virus through an otherwise innocuous visit of a friend or family member or even from interaction with an infected caregiver.[54] Hence, nursing homes and long-term care facilities represent an ideal target to implement and sustain large-scaled testing to reduce the overall severity of COVID-19 and other infectious diseases. Such locations are not unique, but they are revealing—they point to ways that testing could be used moving forward as part of an integrative response.

Entrance to a nursing home or long-term care facility (what we will refer to in aggregate as an LTC in this section) represents a key moment in a caring bond: whether visiting a loved one or friend or participating in activities that bring a social element to elders who can become both physically and socially isolated over time. Yet such visits are not without risk—whether the visit of a small chorale group, the volunteer efforts of an Eagle Scout, or a family visit to see Grandma and share a meal in the cafeteria. In each of these situations, someone who is asymptomatically infected (or infected with such a mild case that given their age and health status, it is viewed as nothing more than a slight inconvenience) may inadvertently spread an illness while intending to bring comfort. In that sense, COVID-19 epitomizes the risks associated with asymptomatic and presymptomatic transmission—a risk that is also present with influenza. In an ideal world, preventative steps would be taken to keep driving down the risk of inadvertently introducing a potentially fatal respiratory infection into a vulnerable community. The first step could surely involve testing.[55]

Testing visitors rapidly represents a small inconvenience but can have a significant benefit. Likewise, testing staff and residents on a regular basis helps to layer in practical steps to identify the potential emergence of infections in a LTC setting. We must still recognize that "entry testing" will be imperfect. Entry tests could be administered using rapid antigen tests that deliver test results within minutes. Visitors might not want to test—yet given the vulnerability of LTC populations, the benefits of reducing a potentially severe disease is likely to outweigh the costs. Ideally, knowing someone is negative is informative and empowering: the effective chance that you are infected is markedly lower than the population-level prevalence. And knowing someone is positive would (hopefully) persuade that individual to postpone a visit to a vulnerable community. Of course, such tests come with caveats—both technical and social. The sensitivity of such tests is not 100%; a large majority of (but not all) individuals who are shedding infectious virus will test positive using an antigen assay. And, given ongoing controversy surrounding imposed testing, facilities may decide that they do not want to reengage.

A policy that requires a test before visiting an LTC would certainly meet with resistance. Precisely so, the rationale for the policy must be explained so that caretakers, residents, staff, and visitors understand their shared role in keeping loved ones safe. But such a policy need not be all-or-nothing given that testing does not work alone. A test-to-visit policy could be linked to updated estimates of community spread levels (see the earlier section on increased at-home testing). That is, agreeing on a tolerable level of risk that an individual is infected in a community could help inform decision-making about when a test-to-visit policy is required as part of layered interventions (e.g., along with an improved airflow infrastructure and mask-wearing). Considering what is at stake, such decisions should be made in light of the cumulative evidence. Nationwide, in the first year of the pandemic, about one-third of total COVID-19 fatalities were in LTCs, despite representing a small fraction of the total number of documented cases.[56] Testing could also help keep the focus of visits on care and joy, rather than fear of spreading a potentially fatal infection. In certain cases, the continued use of masks may be necessary, especially when visiting medically vulnerable individuals. Even then, we must also acknowledge the human desire to see each other, to connect, and to want a normal experience, not one where medical safety overshadows all else. Opening windows and improving indoor air quality are other ways to create a safer environment and more meaningful connections.

This idea of using testing to foster safer interactions has been tried—largely in Europe through variations of a "health pass." The purpose of the health pass was, ostensibly, to reduce the risk of inadvertent spread from asymptomatically infected individuals in public settings. In order to drive acceptance, health passes were often required to access long-distance trains, commercial planes, and restaurants.[57] But such access restrictions had limits. In France, there was no restriction on access to buses, the metro, supermarkets, and the beloved boulangerie, irrespective of vaccination status. The health pass was popular initially, although it was also met with significant resistance, protests, and even clashes between protestors and police.[58] (Keep in mind that protests are far more commonplace in France than in the United States.)

The primary aim of the health pass worked: it incentivized vaccination, because being vaccinated had a halo effect. It opened up more public spaces to individuals with the rapid presentation of a QR code on one's phone. But even such health passes are imperfect, especially with the emergence of variants (particularly Omicron) that have infected previously vaccinated individuals at high rates. Although such post-vaccination infections are milder than outcomes in individuals infected for the first time in the absence of a vaccine, they indicate that vaccinated individuals can be infected and may become unwitting asymptomatic carriers. For this reason, testing can become a way to participate in certain activities at certain times (e.g., when there is high community spread), whether formally (e.g., to visit a nursing home) or informally (e.g., by request of someone hosting a party or gathering). These point-of-interaction testing modes represent an effort to provide information as needed, and then adjust accordingly.

Perhaps one thinks that such point-of-care testing is overwrought. Why test in certain locations when so many parts of society are not testing? Yet shouldn't those who want to test have access to real-time information that could reduce their risk of infection? We do not always know the context for such requests and whether someone may be immunocompromised or have risk factors particularly associated with elevated mortality if exposed and infected. Empathetic reasoning can lead to safer interactions and, in the end, more of the very interactions we crave. In certain circumstances, the collective risk may simply be too high, and new standards will have to evolve so that safe air becomes a prerequisite for interactions, in the same way that we do not want lead in our water or *E. coli* in our beef. Transparency in data collection through testing at the community scale and at points of interaction can become a means to support both public health and socioeconomic outcomes. There is one critical step left, however.

This book's premise has been that asymptomatic spread is a double-edge sword: a silent or mild outcome for some that can lead, inadvertently, to far greater numbers of severe cases for the population as a whole. Yet this premise rests on the presumption that there is an approximately equal balance between asymptomatic and symptomatic cases. If, instead, the fraction of asymptomatic cases could be increased, then COVID-19 outcomes could start to resemble a mild virus, ideally something akin to the common cold or, in a somewhat worse (but not the worst) outcome, something like seasonal influenza. Such an outcome means that asymptomatic spread becomes closer to an endpoint rather than a gateway to failure. One path toward such asymptomatic outcomes was pursued from the start: large-scale, effective vaccination.[59]

CHAPTER 6

Vaccination Requires More than Vaccines

The Miracle of mRNA Vaccines

We have witnessed a miracle. SARS-CoV-2 was first identified in December 2019. The first whole genome sequenced was released on January 9, 2020, through a global sharing initiative intended to facilitate responses to emerging epidemics.[1] Immediately, researchers worldwide began to evaluate the potential for development of vaccines using distinct delivery platforms. Of these, the mRNA-based vaccines have emerged as both the most flexible, changeable, and effective in reducing severe outcomes in vaccinated individuals.[2] Yet the purpose of vaccination is often misunderstood. Vaccination helps those who are vaccinated. It also helps those who are not vaccinated. The former is a kind of personal protection. The latter forms the basis for population-scale immunity. Hence, vaccination helps both the vaccinated and those around them who may not be able to be vaccinated (because of age or eligibility) or who do not elicit strong immune responses to vaccination (potentially because of confounding immune disorders) or have not yet been vaccinated (because of limitations in availability).

The scale of vaccination in the United States and globally is truly extraordinary.[3] In less than a year, multiple public–private partnerships, including the one between the National Institutes of Health (NIH) and Moderna, as well as private companies leveraging the results of publicly funded research (including Pfizer, Johnson & Johnson, and AstraZeneca) identified the key part of the virus that could help train an immune system to ward off future infections, developed prototype vaccines, initiated clinical trials, demonstrated high levels of vaccine safety and efficacy, and then scaled up production so that more than 650 million doses were administered in the United States as of March 2023, a little more than two years after becoming available to the general public. Globally, as of March 2023, more than 13 billion viral doses had been administered, and more than 72% of the world's population had received at least one dose.[4]

This scaling up of vaccine delivery has had a tremendous impact. For those who are vaccinated, the risks of severe infection and fatalities have been reduced by 95% or more.[5] This is a game changer. Particularly in older adults, sustained reduction of fatalities by 95% would at least return expected deaths from COVID-19 to levels comparable to that of seasonal influenza. We should recognize the incredible personal protection that vaccines (especially mRNA-based vaccines) now offer.

Yet more must be done.

There are approximately 8 billion of us on this planet. It would take 16 billion doses to ensure that everyone received a full course of a mRNA vaccine and more than 32 billion to ensure that all received a full primary sequence, primary booster, and second booster. By counts alone, it would seem that we were nearly halfway to this goal as of mid-2023. Yet like many things in public health, the benefits of investment and infrastructure are rarely equally distributed.

Globally, there are significant differences in the distribution of life-saving vaccines. As of March 2022, in South Africa, there was approximately one dose delivered for every two people. The vaccine distribution was even worse in Nigeria, where one dose was administered for every eight people. These low distribution rates contrast with countries in Western Europe—for example, in Spain and Portugal, 85% and 91% of the population, respectively, were vaccinated at the same time.[6] The consequences of such different levels are many. First, fewer vaccinations mean that more individuals are vulnerable to infections and severe outcomes. Second, on aggregate, continued spread in unvaccinated populations can drive the replication of viral variants that may be the grist for evolutionary change that could spill back into better vaccinated countries—leading to the onset of new waves.[7]

If we are to look for differences in vaccination coverage, we do not necessarily need to go abroad. We can find such differences in the United States.

Overall, despite the availability of free and safe vaccines that have been shown to be offer significant protection against severe disease, only two out of three Americas were fully vaccinated as of spring 2022.[8] This means that one in three remained unvaccinated—or more than 100 million individuals (excluding the very young who were not yet eligible to receive the vaccine). That is an unvaccinated population larger than the populations of England, France, Germany, Spain, or Italy. At the earliest stages, the differences in vaccination rates were strongly influenced by race and ethnicity—with Blacks and Hispanics having lower rates of vaccination than non-Hispanic whites.[9] Yet there is another, perhaps even stronger driver of differences in vaccination rates that has grown over time: political identity. In essence, areas with more right-leaning constituents have significantly lower rates of primary COVID-19 vaccine and booster uptake than areas with more moderate or left-leaning constituents. This difference can be seen in figure 6.1.

The conflation of political identity with attitudes toward vaccination has real-world consequences. Beginning in April 2021, the rates of vaccination in counties (and indeed, in states) that voted for Donald Trump lagged behind rates of vaccinations (and states) that voted for Joseph Biden. The overall difference increased with time such that by September 2021, more than 50% of individuals in Biden-supporting counties were vaccinated while less than 40% of individuals in Trump-supporting counties were vaccinated (similar results held through early 2022).[10] The bottom five states in terms of vaccination rates in early 2022 were Alabama, Wyoming, Mississippi, Louisiana, and Idaho (all of which had less than 53% of residents fully vaccinated). The top five states in terms of vaccination rates were Rhode Island, Vermont, Maine, Connecticut, and Massachusetts (all of which had more than 75% residents fully vaccinated). In essence, the top-performing states

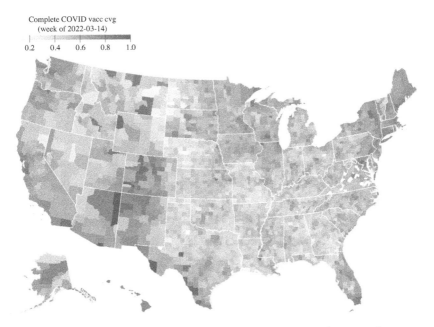

Figure 6.1. Differences in vaccination rates as of March 14, 2022. The rates of vaccination are typically higher in areas associated with moderate or left-leaning constituencies (darker shades). *Source*: Vaccination map courtesy of Shweta Bansal, Georgetown University, following methods described in Tu, A., et al. (2022). Characterizing the spatiotemporal heterogeneity of the COVID-19 vaccination landscape. *American Journal of Epidemiology* 191: 1792–1802. https://doi.org/10.1093/aje/kwac080

in the United States had vaccination rates similar to that of Germany while the bottom-performing states had vaccination rates similar to that of Venezuela, Bangladesh, Bolivia, Tunisia, and Russia.[11]

These differences have consequences. But to unpack the consequences and to devise better approaches to protect individuals and populations requires a consideration of the principles by which vaccines work—not just for the vaccinated, but for the community in which they are embedded. We can do so by turning again to simple models of the impact of vaccines at the individual to population levels. In chapter 3, a simplified model was used to connect the spread of disease among individuals with or without symptoms to population-level effects. The outcome was striking: the most severe outcomes at the population scale occurred when there was an intermediate level of asymptomatic infections at the individual scale. This same kind of mechanistic structure can be used to provide the rationale for why vaccines can be effective and why they help both the individual who is vaccinated and the community at large.

How Vaccination Curbs Epidemic Spread

In order to understand the potential benefits of vaccination, we need to consider how the vaccination status of individuals ends up protecting others—including others who may not yet be vaccinated or are not able to receive a vaccine. As explained in part 1, infectious individuals can come into contact with susceptible individuals leading to new infections. These infectious individuals may then recover. Recovered individuals are presumed to have increased immunity to future infections and increased likelihood that reinfections will not lead to severe disease. But, vaccination provides a safer route to immunity. The question, then, becomes: Can a sufficiently broad vaccine campaign protect even those who remain unvaccinated? The answer is yes. Rather than starting with a simplified epidemiological model, let us instead turn to historical data (figure 6.2).

The figure shows the intensity of spread from more than 25 states in the United States in the decades leading up to and after the introduction of measles vaccines. The change is dramatic and stark—and consistent with other viral infections, including polio. Before the introduction of the polio vaccine, the incidence was typically on the order of 200 new cases of polio per 100,000 individuals in the United States. In modern terms, because polio tends to affect the young (e.g., children under 10 years of age), this is equivalent to avoiding 100,000 total polio cases per year. Instead, polio nearly vanished from the United States by the 1960s and was effectively eliminated by 1979. No more. Unfortunately, the Centers for Disease Control (CDC) issued a national alert after detecting circulating poliovirus in Rockland County, New York, in fall 2022.[12] The polio vaccine uses an inactive form of the virus, providing immunity to those who receive it. But, this inactivated

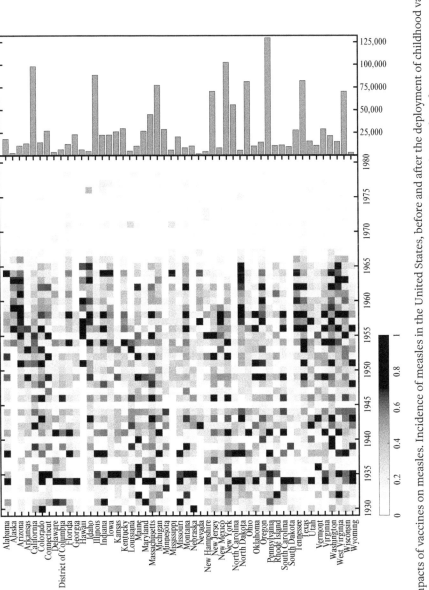

Figure 6.2. Impacts of vaccines on measles. Incidence of measles in the United States, before and after the deployment of childhood vaccines in 1963 (left). States are listed on rows. Columns denote the year. The darkness of shading indicates the number of cases per 100,000 relative to a state's maximum number. The solid line denotes the time of vaccine introduction (right). The bar graph depicts the maximum number of measles cases in a given state in a given year in the range shown. *Source:* Reproduced from figure 12.8 of Weitz, J.S. (2024) *Quantitative Biosciences: Dynamics Across Cells, Organisms, and Populations.* Princeton University Press.

virus can sometimes replicate in immunocompromised individuals or in nonimmunized individuals, reacquiring genetic mutations that can allow it to spread and cause paralysis or death. Low levels of community vaccination compound this problem and can lead to an outbreak.

The decline in measles in the United States as shown in figure 6.2 has followed a similar pattern to that of polio. Although there are occasional measles outbreaks, the incidence has remained far lower than it was before the widespread introduction of vaccines. Measles outbreaks are often linked to overseas travel and then amplified in communities with low vaccination rates. Again, drops in community vaccination rates increase the risk of outbreaks. Public health efforts to increase the childhood measles vaccination rate have helped communities with low vaccination rates respond to severe measles outbreaks (more on this shortly). Thankfully, vaccination coverage remains above 90% nationwide for the majority of recommended childhood vaccines—including the MMR vaccine (measles, mumps, and rubella).[13]

These examples illustrate the power of vaccines in providing immunity safely. In contrast to infection-derived immunity, vaccines can be used to protect individuals and their communities from the devastating effects of illnesses that affect children and adults. But there is one more piece to the puzzle to understand the rapid reduction in disease incidence in just a few years after the introduction of childhood vaccines in the United States.

> *The lesson:* Most individuals (but not every individual) must be vaccinated for (nearly) every individual to receive the protective benefits of vaccines.

To understand the power of vaccines to help the individual and those they interact with, consider the situation where an infectious individual might typically infect 3 others in a population where everyone else is susceptible. Figure 6.3 contrasts the spread of an infection in an entirely susceptible population with the case where there is a disease spreading in a population where 2 of 3 individuals have been vaccinated.

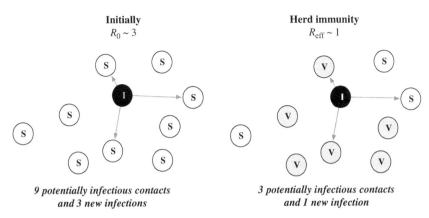

Initially
$R_0 \sim 3$

Herd immunity
$R_{\text{eff}} \sim 1$

9 potentially infectious contacts
and 3 new infections

3 potentially infectious contacts
and 1 new infection

Figure 6.3. Contrast of the spread of a disease in an entirely susceptible population (left) versus a partially vaccinated population (right). In both cases, there are nine contacts, of which three could lead to an infection in the absence of vaccines (left) but only one new infection when two of the three are vaccinated. Here, disease status can be susceptible (S), infectious (I), or vaccinated (V). This image does not include the transition to a recovered state (R).

As was already described, if one person is infected and typically infects 3 others, this can lead to exponential spread. The 3 newly infected people go on to infect 9 more, and then 27, and soon the numbers grow fast—exponentially so—leading to a large-scale outbreak. But instead, imagine that 2 out of every 3 people in a community were vaccinated. In that case, a single infectious individual would still come into contact with others. But of the 3 potentially infectious contacts, perhaps 2 of 3 would have been vaccinated, thereby reducing the number of infections from 3 to 1. Hence, instead of the disease growing in number, the average number of cases in the next "generation" is expected to be the same. As previously infected individuals recover, the average number of infections at the individual levels drops below 1. This means that the population number of infections drops as well. Rather than the disease proliferating, a sufficiently vaccinated community is far more likely to experience a small cluster of cases rather than a full-fledged outbreak. Moreover, if the vaccination rate were to increase (e.g., to 80%), then it is likely that a single infectious individual would not infect anyone at all, because each of the 3 people they would have infected would already be vaccinated. Hence, when a single unvaccinated child returns from an international trip with measles, that child would almost certainly not infect others.

Vaccine-derived population immunity means that it is far more difficult for cases to increase in number. So, even if some individuals are not vaccinated, they still get a protective benefit, because paths that a virus might take to reach them have been cut off, short-circuited by the vaccine. This is a very different outcome than in the case of *herd immunity* acquired through the mass accumulation of infections and, for the survivors, of infection-derived immunity. This is yet another benefit of vaccine-derived rather than infection-derived immunity at population scales. The herd immunity threshold can be reached with vaccines *before* an infection is widespread. In contrast, infections are expected to be at their maximum value when herd immunity is reached because of the accumulation of infection and recovery events. As a result, even though infections begin to go down, there are still many more individuals who will be infected. This concept of epidemic overshot was discussed in chapter 3. Large-scale vaccination stops overshoot because it works to prevent a case or case cluster from becoming an outbreak. The rare introduction of an infectious case does not lead to more cases, so the disease does not take off in the first place.

The fact that vaccines also protect those who do not get vaccinated reveals a potential vulnerability. What happens if someone begins to think, "Why should I get vaccinated if I perceive there is some risk of the vaccine and if enough people around me get vaccinated?" This problem has grown ever more pressing because of coordinated efforts to spread false and misleading information on the potential harms of vaccines.

Typically, public health officials aim for vaccination levels of 95% or above for most childhood diseases when stopping transmission is the goal (i.e., exceeding the expected herd immunity threshold). This vaccination rate is grounded in the simplified image shown in figure 6.3. Measles is highly transmissible and infects ~15 other individuals within unvaccinated communities. As a result, the herd immunity threshold occurs when only 1/15 individuals remains susceptible, equivalent to vaccinating 95% or more of a population to reach vaccine-derived herd immunity. Once the vaccination rates drop below those levels, bad things can happen.

From Marin County and Beyond

Marin County, California, provides an example of the challenge in confronting vaccination gaps in the United States—and ways in which anti-vaccination hubs defy simplified conservative-or-liberal dichotomies. Marin County is located north of San Francisco and is connected to the city by the Golden Gate Bridge. It is a decidedly left-leaning county. Biden received more than 80% of the presidential vote in 2020. Yet, Marin County has experienced multiple, severe measles outbreaks. The reason? Not enough kids had been vaccinated, and suspected international travel introduced measles into a community that was only partially vaccinated.

Conventional explanations for COVID-19 vaccine hesitancy tend to frame the issue in terms of political affiliation—with surveys revealing that individuals who identify as Republicans are less likely to be vaccinated than those who identify as Democrats.[14,15] Yet, the reasons for vaccine hesitancy are complex and include a mix of personal, socioeconomic, and religious reasons—and these reasons can change with time.[16] In the case of Marin County, previous hesitancy to the MMR vaccine series was fueled by medical mistrust often allied with otherwise liberal-leaning politics.[17] This mistrust was accelerated by discredited reports of a link between vaccines and autism.[18] In the absence of sufficient community-wide vaccination levels, measles can spread within (partially) unvaccinated households, leading to an increased risk for those children still too young to receive the three-dose series. There were significant measles outbreaks in Marin County in 2015[19] and in the Bay area in 2018.[20] The backlash was significant. Given widespread recognition that measles outbreaks were still possible, Marin County public health officials launched a systematic campaign to increase vaccination rates, leading to county-level rates exceeding 94% of incoming kindergarten students by fall 2019 (the highest ever recorded for the county—and close to, but still below, the statewide average).[21]

This cycle reveals the potential for oscillations in the ways that individuals may consciously or unconsciously game vaccination requirements.[22] In the event that everyone complies, then one can derive a benefit from not vaccinating—because the protection is enabled by the decisions of others. Yet, if many begin to think that same way, then community-wide vaccination rates decline, and the risk of an outbreak increases, eventually to a critical level. At this point, then the natural reaction is to recognize that there is no longer a population-derived benefit, and it is imperative to get vaccinated to gain personal protection against a spreading virus. Over time, as immunity increases, the risk of recurring outbreaks goes down, and then the incentive not to vaccinate increases—and not for the first time: individuals acting in their own self-interest can generate worse outcomes than had they acted cooperatively.[23] These kinds of cycles of behavior[24] are also relevant to the efforts to deploy COVID-19 vaccines at population scales.

COVID-19 vaccines were introduced in early 2020, and they were made available at first to the elderly and those in higher-risk and front-line worker categories. This choice was intended to deploy a limited resource to individuals who were likely to derive the biggest personal benefit. The increase in severity and fatalities with age all point to the need to rapidly vaccinate the old (and those with known risk factors) as a means to reduce the worst outcomes—these outcomes also overwhelm hospitals and intensive care units (ICUs), making it harder to obtain basic and emergency care. Yet, for many reasons, vaccination rates among the old varied significantly. As noted earlier in this chapter, vaccination rates varied widely between "red" and "blue" states, with gaps in coverage exceeding 10% or more and persisting into early 2022.[25] This meant that far too many people remained vulnerable to infection, even as the Delta wave and eventually the Omicron wave spread throughout the United States.

Sadly, the majority of the hundreds of thousands of fatalities from COVID-19 in 2021 were preventable—with the risk of dying from COVID-19 being 12 to 25 times higher for unvaccinated individuals compared to vaccinated individuals.[26] Many hundreds of thousands of older adults died of COVID-19 in 2021. Moreover, there was even a slight shift to younger ages in fatalities because many older adults did get vaccinated and many middle-aged adults did not. In 2020, there were ~230,000 fatalities in those age 75 and older and ~130,000 fatalities in those 50 to 74 years of age. In 2021, there were ~205,000 fatalities in those age 75 and up and ~150,000 fatalities in those 50 to 74 years of age. Although 2022 was not as severe as previous years, the United States experienced more than 250,000 documented COVID-19 fatalities, far less than had vaccines not been available but far more than had vaccines been adopted nearly universally among adults—especially vulnerable older adults.[27] Beyond the missed opportunity to vaccinate more of the US population, the gaps in global vaccination are even more startling[28]—and a topic for the action opportunity section at the end of this chapter.

What Do Vaccines Stop? (and Why It Matters)

The COVID-19 vaccines, including those of Pfizer, NIH-Moderna, Johnson & Johnson, and AstraZeneca, were all subjected to a systematic series of clinical trials meant to evaluate safety, then efficacy (in a small subject population), and then efficacy again (albeit in a far larger population). But in all cases the objective of the trial was to make a measurable impact on severe disease. All of the vaccines were shown to significant improve outcomes in terms of the reduction in *symptomatic* infections. Figure 6.4 presents a summary of results published in late 2020 in the *New England Journal of Medicine* (perhaps the most venerated medical journal in the United States)—although the data itself had been available to regulators many months before.

The figure shows a comparison of the cumulative incidence of COVID-19 in the study population when comparing outcomes in individuals given a placebo (the top gray curve) against outcomes in individuals given the Pfizer mRNA vaccine (also known as BNT162b2; the bottom black curve). The placebo and vaccine curves nearly coincide for the first 7 to 10 days after the first dose. This means it takes some time for protective benefits to emerge. The second dose was then given at day 21. From there, the evidence is clear: the placebo

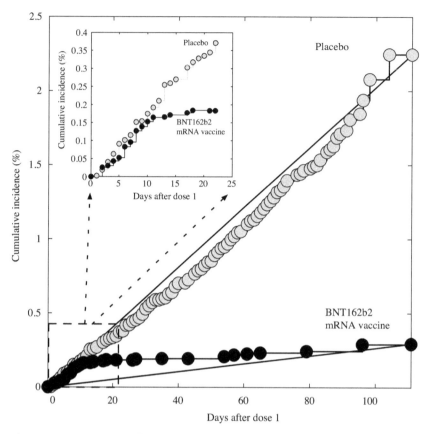

Figure 6.4. Comparative effectiveness of the Pfizer-BioNTech BNT162b2 mRNA vaccine versus a placebo. The x-axis is days after the first dose; the y-axis compares the cumulative incidence of symptomatic COVID-19. The gray line with gray circles denotes the placebo cohort, and the solid line with black circles denotes the vaccine-treated cohort. The inset image focuses in on the first 22 days of the comparison, while the main plot includes data beyond 100 days. In total, 43,448 individuals received injections, 21,720 with the mRNA vaccine and 21,728 with the placebo. As is apparent, there is a significant difference in outcome between vaccine and placebo recipients. *Source*: Redrawn from data in figure 3 of Polack, F.P., et al. (2020). Safety and efficacy of the BNT162b2 mRNA Covid-19 vaccine. *New England Journal of Medicine* 383: 2603–2615. https://doi.org/10.1056/NEJMoa2034577.

incidence continues its steady march upward, wholly unlike the incidence within the vaccinated group. Statistical analysis reveals that the vaccine is extremely protective against symptomatic infection—with estimates of protection between 90–98%. Yet, every study comes with limitations. This one did, too. As the authors noted, one of the key remaining questions was whether or not "the vaccine protects against asymptomatic infection and transmission to unvaccinated persons."

Hence, for all the effectiveness of the vaccine against symptomatic COVID-19, severe disease, and fatalities, it was not clear if the vaccine was also able to completely protect against infection. Perhaps vaccinated individuals would still become infected, albeit with mild or asymptomatic cases, and could then pass on an infection to others. The fact that many did get infected—often with mild or asymptomatic cases—became a central counterargument to suggest that the vaccines did not work. This difference sits at the core of vaccine campaigns and intent. We must address the consequences when a vaccine protects against severe disease versus the case when it protects against infection entirely. If we do not address the potential for individuals to be infected with milder (or even asymptomatic) cases post-vaccine, then we once again have missed the opportunity to develop effective public health strategies, and we risk confusing the public with misplaced expectations of what the vaccine can and cannot do.

The promise of vaccines was (and is) that they will end the pandemic. And there are at least some historical precedents for such an impact. The stories of the measles and polio vaccines are remarkable. In countries where childhood vaccination is nearly universal, these illnesses have in fact largely disappeared. But the battle to eliminate COVID-19 was always going to be difficult because of the speed and scope of spread—particularly because of the ability of the virus to spread even when it did not induce symptoms. The chance that vaccines would be able to be deployed effectively was entirely unclear. It remains remarkable that vaccines were developed, evaluated, verified for safety and efficacy, and then scaled up so that billions of doses could be produced, distributed, and administered within a year after the first sequences of SARS-CoV-2 were available. The story of how COVID-19 vaccines were developed has been covered extensively in short-form,[29] feature,[30] and book-length reporting.[31,32] This coverage includes the necessary prework on mRNA delivery platforms (as but one example), rapid sequencing, choice of a target,[33] and the insights learned from ongoing work to scale up coronavirus vaccine platforms to meet a global need.

There are other cases where the efficacy of vaccines is not nearly as profound. A vaccine may not completely halt disease spread for multiple reasons, including (i) weakening of a vaccine-derived immune response over time[34] and (ii) virus evolution, such that new variants escape the ability of the immune system to identify and eliminate them.[35] Influenza vaccines are notoriously hit-or-miss. In a good year, they might offer a reduction of the risk of infection of approximately 60%, but often they fare far worse.[36] The results of the COVID-19 vaccine trials suggested that large-scale protection was possible if nearly everyone who was eligible to be vaccinated was vaccinated. Like for measles, the estimated value of the basic reproduction number (R_0) provided a rationale for the levels of vaccination required to stop the spread. If R_0 for COVID-19 was 3, then perhaps or 67% of the population would need to be vaccinated to reach vaccine-derived herd immunity. If R_0 was higher (whether for the historical strain or variants), then it could take 75% (if R_0 was 4) or 80% of the population (if R_0 was 5), or even higher, to reach vaccine-derived herd immunity. This link between the strength of spread and the level of vaccination required to stop an outbreak underlies the rationale for Dr. Anthony Fauci's comments as a member of the White House Coronavirus Task Force in late 2020 that "50% would have to get vaccinated before you start to see an impact" and "75 to 85% would have to get vaccinated if you want to have that blanket of herd immunity."[37] But vaccinating children to protect against measles when the vast majority of adults are already vaccinated presents very different epidemiological challenges than vaccinating a population, many of whom have already been infected, in the midst of a global outbreak. Furthermore, even minimum estimates for protective population-level coverage are based on models of pathogens for which a single exposure, either through vaccination or infection, leads to long-lasting immunity. This turned out not to be the case for COVID-19.

It takes time to get hundreds of millions of individuals vaccinated. In practice, the United States has lagged behind much of the developed world in terms of vaccination rates. This means that the pace of vaccination can take as long as a wave—if not two waves—of infections for large enough levels of vaccination to blunt the impact. Moreover, even if one observes an impact, there is no counterfactual to compare to (outside of model scenarios). How would we know if things could be worse? The link between plateaus and declines in cases and changes in perception can often mean that changes in behavior are connected to reductions in epidemic prevalence, even if the relaxation of restrictions tends to lead to an increase in transmission. The cycling in and out of waves can generate fatigue among individuals who no longer perceive a risk or see the point of continuing to worry about COVID-19.

But in spring 2021, there was a sense of optimism. Safe and effective vaccines were available to every American who wanted one—and they were free.

Failure to Vaccinate

Vaccines represented a chance to systematically protect hundreds of millions of people in America and many billions globally. For the first time since lockdowns a year before, there seemed to be a path out of the pandemic. The number of vaccine doses administered rose steadily from hundreds of thousands of doses a day in early January (primarily targeted to the old, severely at risk, and frontline medical workers) to more than 3 million doses administered per day by mid-April 2021.[38] The demand for vaccines was intense and not always met. Reports of "line skipping" to secure a vaccine were rampant,[39] as were efforts to communicate the rationale for waiting in line and what the line was supposed to do (i.e., serve the most vulnerable, health care workers, and the immunocompromised and elderly before younger, healthier individuals).[40] But is it unethical to line skip or drive to another state to get a vaccine if vaccine demand was in fact heterogeneous?[41] Indeed, by July 4, 2021, the levels of vaccine administration had dropped down to less than 1 million a day. It was often hard to find someone who was willing to get vaccinated, even if the overall vaccination rates meant that less than 50% of the eligible population was fully vaccinated in time for Independence Day celebrations. Consequently, instead of a summer 2021 exit from COVID-19, there was another wave.

The wave became the proof needed by vaccine skeptics to reinforce their claims that vaccines did not work. The argument goes that if vaccines are so effective and so many have already been vaccinated, then how is it possible for there to be nearly as many fatalities as before? Moreover, in states with poor vaccinations, then the absence of an even stronger wave can become more evidence that vaccines are not protective. And each instance of someone being reinfected becomes yet another example to build a narrative that vaccines do not work—and perhaps that they do more harm than good. Let us unwrap and address each of these arguments in term.

Critique 1: How can a wave be strong when so many have been vaccinated?

Vaccines have a demonstrated impact in reducing disease severity, with large-scale trials showing an ~95% decrease in risk of severe infection with respect to historical strains. If the mid-April rate of more than 3 million doses administered per day had been sustained for three more months, then the United States would have been on track to vaccinate nearly the entire US adult population. Yet, by July 4, 2021, less than half of US adults had been fully vaccinated—while children remained wholly unvaccinated. This means that more than half of adults remained unvaccinated at the start of the Delta wave. As a result, a large section of the population did not receive the protective benefits of the vaccine. This fact, combined with the emergence of the more infectious Delta variant, meant that more than 150 million individuals in the United States remained unvaccinated—including nearly all children—providing ample opportunities for spread. Moreover, if the impression is that the vaccine will provide herd immunity, then individuals may begin to do things they would not have done had they not been protected (e.g., going to restaurants and spending time indoors without masks). But with so many unvaccinated individuals remaining, the spread of an infection from a mild or asymptomatic case can generate more infections (including severe cases) in others.

Critique 2: Why aren't waves always as strong in states with poor vaccination levels?

As of July 4, 2021, there had been more than 30 million documented COVID-19 cases in the United States.[42] But such case counts were a significant underestimate of the true cumulative impact—for reasons already explained in the first part of this book. Asymptomatic infections and under-testing meant that most cases were not documented, likely approaching a rate of four to five actual cases per each documented case. As a result, 30 million documented cases likely represented more than 120 million prior infections. This means that a substantial fraction of individuals in United States had either been infected and/or vaccinated by mid-2021 in contrast to early 2020, when the population was almost entirely immunologically naive. How can we estimate how much immunity is from vaccines and how much is from getting infected? We cannot simply add these two numbers together; for example, if 60% of individuals had been infected and 60% had been vaccinated, that does not mean 120% of people have been infected or vaccinated. Instead, we categorize individuals as (i) previously infected, not vaccinated; (ii) vaccinated, not previously infected; (iii) both vaccinated and previously infected; (iv) immunologically naive. By accounting for these four possibilities, we can estimate the total population immunity at a focal level (e.g., county or state), recognizing that individuals who have already been infected are also significantly less likely to be infected and, if infected, to have a severe case. This means that there are many ways to get similar levels of population immunity.

For example, a state with 75% of the population vaccinated and 20% of the population having been infected may have a similar level of individuals who are no longer immunologically naive as does a population with 45% vaccinated and 60% previously vaccinated. Such significant variations were in fact commonplace in the United States as of mid-2021; they represent the difference between a state like Vermont (well vaccinated, with a limited number of cumulative infection) versus one like South Dakota (poorly vaccinated, with many cumulative infections). As a result, at a certain point, a poorly vaccinated state may not experience a significant new wave if it already (and fairly recently) had large-scale infections. Population immunity is real—but reaching it through vaccine-derived immunity is far safer. In fact, increasing evidence suggests that the greatest protective benefits is associated with "hybrid" immunity—the immunity derived from having been vaccinated and also been infected, hopefully in that order.[43,44] Hybrid immunity is likely far more common than recognized precisely because of the extent of asymptomatic and undocumented infections. According to the CDC, the United States passed 20 million documented cases in the first week of 2021.[45] Assuming a 4:1 or 5:1 ratio of actual cases per documented cases, however, suggests that more than 80 million or 100 million individuals were already infected before the Delta wave began.

Critique 3: Why should folks get vaccinated when vaccinated individuals can still get infected?

The promise of vaccines are twofold: (i) they might halt the spread of a disease entirely if vaccination levels pass critical levels, and (ii) they might turn a deadly disease into a mild one. For COVID-19, the first promise has not and will not be realized, certainly not anytime soon. Not only have vaccination levels not reached critical levels, but vaccinated individuals can still be infected more likely with mild/asymptomatic outcomes and potential transmit to others. Recall that in chapter 3, we learned how an intermediate level of asymptomatic spread can, paradoxically, lead to increases in population-level fatalities. Yet, if the asymptomatic rates gets even higher, then at some point the cumulative fatalities are expected to decrease. If it is a purely asymptomatic infection (or one that is sufficiently mild/subclinical) then it is unlikely to cause fatalities. This is similar to the common cold. This is why folks should get vaccinated. If enough individuals are vaccinated, then even if they become infected they are more likely to have a mild rather than a severe cases; and finally, from a population perspective, reduction in severe cases leads to better care for those who need it and less need for blanket restrictions.

Unfortunately, we observed a clarion example of how vaccination policies affect countries with presumably similar levels of population immunity during the concurrent Omicron waves in Hong Kong and New Zealand in early 2022. Both countries had previously had zero-COVID policies and imposed severe travel restrictions, and yet in New Zealand, the vaccination rates (including boosters) for older individuals were far higher than in Hong Kong. The differences in outcomes are stark. While both countries have seen similar levels of cases, Hong Kong experienced a significantly higher death rate with a case fatality rate of 4.7%, while New Zealand had a case fatality rate of 0.1%. The likely reason: in New Zealand, 98% of those age 80 and older were fully vaccinated, whereas only 34% of those 80 and older in Hong Kong were fully vaccinated.[46] The take-home message is important:

> Vaccination makes a dramatic difference in severe outcomes, even if it cannot fully stop the spread of disease.

All of these arguments suggest that vaccination at scale and particularly among vulnerable populations is critical to protect a population from severe outcomes, to reduce fatalities, and to safeguard hospital resources. But, in the United States, such paths have not been taken equally, with gaps that began in spring 2021 persisting even now. These gaps have consequences.

There are many ways to build up immunity in a population. But, in early 2021, when vaccinations became widely available, all US states (and their governors) faced a challenge: how to increase vaccination rates to increase the number of individuals who were no longer immunologically naive. The objective was to reduce incidence and, even more importantly, to reduce disease burden and fatalities (figure 6.5).

In February 2021, the United States passed a grim milestone: more than 500,000 confirmed deaths from COVID-19.[47] Yet, there was also a sense of hope. mRNA vaccines were widely available and could potentially blunt the impact of the pandemic's spread. But, to do so, many

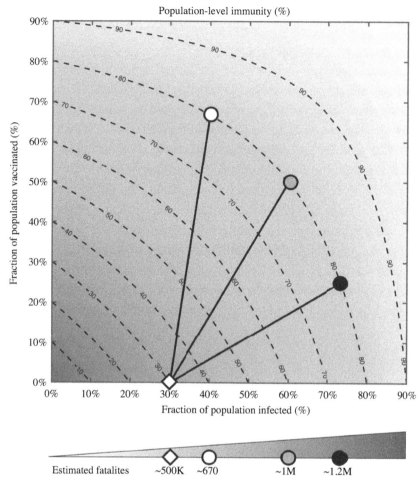

Figure 6.5. Potential trajectories of vaccination campaigns starting with approximately 30% of the population infected and approximately 500,000 fatalities. The x-axis shows the fraction of the population infected, and the y-axis shows the fraction of the population vaccinated. Assuming that vaccination and infection are independent leads to a set of equivalent combinations of infection and vaccination levels (the dashed contour lines, equivalent to the percentage chance that a random individual was infected, vaccinated, or both). The three scenarios denote trajectories in moving from a population that has ~30% infected (diamond) to those with high (white circle), intermediate (gray circle), and low (black circle) levels of vaccination. Each of these scenarios reaches 80% population immunity, albeit with very different levels of infection (x-axis) and estimated fatalities (scale bar at the bottom), which are proportional to cumulative infections. *Source*: Adapted from Lopman, B.A., et al. (2021). A framework for monitoring population immunity to SARS-CoV-2. *Annals of Epidemiology* 63: 75–78. https://doi.org/10.1016/j.annepidem.2021.08.013.

people had to be vaccinated—quickly. Figure 6.5 captures this moment in time through a contour plot of the ways in which a population builds up immunity through a combination of infections (the x-axis) and/or vaccinations (the y-axis). Achieving a "blanket" level of protection requires moving the population immunity level to approximately 80%. Yet the initial level was in fact far higher than widely appreciated. Because of asymptomatic infections, we estimated that approximately 30% of the United States had already been infected by February 2021, or approximately 100 million total infections—four to five times higher than the reported case number. This means that there was in fact a substantial number of individuals who were no longer immunologically naive. This population immunity came with incredible costs—from fatalities, orphaned children, hospitalizations, intubations, and the lingering impacts of severe disease (including long COVID).

The question, then, is how could states drive policy and vaccination campaigns to move toward an 80% level of population immunity? Because of prior infections, vaccines would inevitably be used both on immunologically naive individuals and those with some immune memory of interacting with SARS-CoV-2. Because of the large number of asymptomatic/mild cases, it was likely that even more vaccinations would need to be administered than if one could preselect those who remained immunologically naive. The three scenarios in figure 6.5 all denote ways to reach 80% population immunity, albeit differently. By vaccinating rapidly, the United States could end up reaching 80% levels (open circle) and potentially with hundreds of thousands fewer fatalities than through an intermediate or poor campaign (the shaded and black circles, respectively). The consequences of each of the choices depends on the cumulative infections, and so the objective of states should have been to move "up" in population immunity through vaccination. In practice, however, we did not and do not know who had been infected. This gap in understanding remains a missed opportunity to leverage the best of vaccines without incurring the costs of promising that they alone will stop the problem.

Systematic surveys to identify who had been infected (via antibody assays) could have been used to characterize the cumulative rates of infection as a means to help project the ongoing population immunity levels before and during vaccination campaigns.[48] If scaled up even further, such assays could have even helped to prioritize who to vaccinate and perhaps could have been used to turn a two-dose series into a single-dose series, contingent on confirmed prior infection. Doing so would have acknowledged that infection-derived immunity has an impact, while communicating that the costs of such immunity are high. Only those who survive the infection have immunity. Hence, we should be able to continue to tell the facts as they are about risk levels and, in doing so, be in a better position to explain the value of vaccines and their limitations when deployed at scale in states with very different pandemic experiences.

Action Opportunity: Building a Resilient Population Immunity

Vaccines are a milestone in public health.[49] They represent the shield protecting our children from the threat of infection from measles, rubella, and polio. Vaccines are also the reason that the death toll from COVID-19 is not even higher. The development and public administration of vaccines in early 2021 has been a resounding success. Yet, despite the widespread availability of vaccines, many tens of millions of Americans have chosen not to be vaccinated. The consequences are grave. Misinformation and vaccine hesitation likely led to more than 240,000 preventable fatalities in the United States alone.[50] Even as tens of millions of Americans rejected free and safe vaccines, billions worldwide had no option to make the choice. Estimates suggest that vaccine-sharing inequity has led to millions of preventable deaths globally.[51] Addressing how the United States collaborates globally will shape future public health priorities.[52]

On the one hand, the incredible speed, safety, and efficacy of mRNA-based vaccines will not be fully realized in the face of pushback and entrenched misinformation that asserts mRNA-based vaccines are a part of a global conspiracy. Like many features of the pandemic response, the vaccine "debate" has revealed that our barriers to a better normal are far from exclusively scientific but are also fundamentally linked to individual behavior, social norms, and the engagement of different communities. Medical mistrust among individuals with awareness and/or direct experience of mistreatment by institutionalized health care can drive vaccine hesitancy. For example, Black participants in a US survey expressed the greatest level of medical mistrust and vaccine hesitancy.[53] What has been surprising to some is the extent to which preferences for vaccination are also influenced by partisanship. Multiple studies reported that self-identified liberals and moderates were more likely than self-identified conservatives to express a willingness to get vaccinated (e.g., as in a May 2020 study conducted prospectively, well-before mRNA vaccines were available).[54] Likewise, multiple studies found that the vaccination gap could be partially explained by political partisanship in precisely the same way as anticipated—with liberals and independents more likely to be vaccinated than conservatives.[55] For example, in April 2021, self-identified Democrats made up 36% of unvaccinated adults in contrast to self-identified Republicans, who made up 43% of vaccinated adults. This gap grew over time. By October 2021, self-identified Democrats made up 17% of unvaccinated adults in contrast to self-identified Republicans, who made up 60% of vaccinated adults. Hence, fewer people remained unvaccinated, but those individuals increasingly identified as Republicans.

If we are to get the most benefit out of vaccines, then we must be willing to share what vaccines can do and what vaccines cannot yet do, and we must invest in infrastructure that goes well beyond the development and trial-based evaluation of vaccines. Large-scale development and manufacturing can ensure that vaccines are available, safe, and effective. That still leaves a major hurdle: getting vaccines into arms. The experience in 2021 and 2022 reveals what public health authorities should have anticipated: getting vaccines into arms, especially more than once, takes far more than technical know-how to build resilient population immunity. It requires finding different ways to go the extra mile to reach the population where they are and to confront the reasons for gaps in vaccination and booster coverage in a complicated and often antagonistic information landscape.[56]

But before discussing how to develop a resilient population immunity, we must first understand where we are.

In January 2020, nearly all 8 billion of us on this planet were effectively immunologically naive with respect to SARS-CoV-2. That is, our immune systems had no memory of an experience with this novel, emerging virus. More than a few years later, the vast majority of humans on this planet have had some direct interactions with the virus. Some of us have been infected, and some of us more than once. Some of us have been vaccinated; some of us more than once. And some of us have been infected and vaccinated. For each of those individuals, the human immune system now has a unique record of signatures that has been imprinted in our immunological memory. This means that we now produce specialized molecules—antibodies—that can potentially neutralize viruses as they circulate in our nasal passages and lungs. In addition, our immune systems will produce a specialized type of immune memory cells—B cells—that circulate in our organs, watching and waiting for signs of a reinvasion and signaling to other cells to join in the defense when needed. In the event that a new exposure happens, then there is a far greater chance that the initial dose of viruses that enter into our lungs are unable to replicate fast enough to overcome the body's defenses. Even if the virus does replicate, the presence of memory B cells helps to speed up the initial response, leading to a more mild course of disease, thereby reducing the risk of a severe infection. Yet—and this is a radically important problem—in the United States. we have little to no idea of each of our experiences with the virus. Because we do not have this information, we are less likely to be able to assess which communities are more vulnerable to severe infections in the event of case increases and in cases where new variants spread that may be able to escape initial detection and clearance based on the immune memory of past interactions.

What would a profile of individual histories with COVID-19 look like? Figure 6.6 provides a snapshot of one type of signature and the

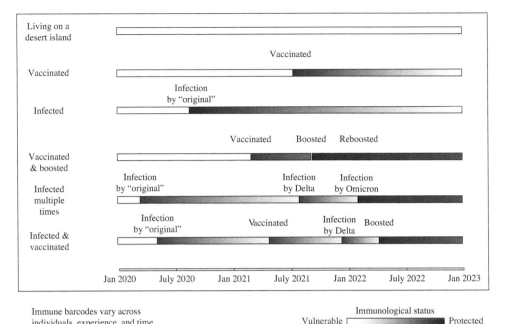

Figure 6.6. Immune barcodes by individuals will vary with prior interactions and time and also shift as a result of changes in the landscape of current variants. The rows are ordered by the approximate relative risk of severe disease at the end of the focal period (here January 2023).

ways in which each of us has experienced COVID-19, focusing only on those who survived infections.

Each of the rows represents an individual, with the shading in the bars presenting an integrated metric of where the individual is, at a given moment, on the spectrum from vulnerable to infected to protected from infection. Each of the rows starts in the vulnerable category, and some stay there for longer. That is, individual behaviors, their environment, and their socioeconomic context (and some luck of the good or bad kind) drove outcomes for the bulk of 2020. Those unlucky enough to be infected and lucky enough to have survived (without lingering complications) would have a postinfection immune memory that could make them protected, if not to infection, then at least to the risk of severe disease. In contrast, individuals who managed to avoid infection remained in the vulnerable status until their first vaccines in 2021. Each of us is different, and our pandemic experiences have been different. These differences mean that we cannot simply rely on a singular event—a single vaccine or a single infection event—and assume that we are now protected.[57] Instead, it will take multiple vaccine doses and recognition that although vaccinations are preferred, our immune memory is shaped by infection, perhaps even more durably than by vaccines. There may even be synergies where a single vaccine dose administered after an infection can produce a durable and protective immune response equivalent to that of two doses in individuals without prior infections.[58] Even these imprints of prior interactions are not permanent because immunity wanes over time, both due to declining levels of circulating antibodies and the evolutionary changes in the virus that make it harder for an immune system to recognize an evolving threat.

Developing a framework for understanding, quantifying, and improving population-level immunity will take a coordination of multiple factors. First, more vaccines need to be administered into arms, not just in the United States but globally. Second, the content of mRNA vaccines likely needs updating so that individuals who receive a booster are not getting more of the same information on the viral protein but something new. The new thing they receive will be a mRNA molecule that encodes information for our own immune cells to recognize circulating variants rather than the original SARS-CoV-2 strain. Third, personalization of responses will require investment in linking immune memory and future risk. This will not be easy, but it is the kind of moonshot investment that the United States should want to take.

Administering vaccines at scale, at home and abroad

The introduction of vaccines in early 2021 heralded a watershed moment in the fight against COVID. But the work is far from done. There is a tremendous gap between having vaccines and getting them into arms. Part of the gap has to do with basic access, information, and trust issues. Vaccination distributions are unlikely to be equitable across the community if a limited number of vaccines are available and one must navigate tiered government websites or try to be the first one to log in and claim a vaccination spot at a local pharmacy. Even when such obstacles are overcome, fundamental concerns about the safety of vaccines may be reflected in communities where historic gaps in treatment and intentional acts of mistreatment have undermined confidence in public health authorities.[59] Precisely this kind of mistrust had lingering effects in early efforts to provide HIV prevention education to the Black community.[60]

There is room for change and even optimism, however. Positive experiences with mRNA vaccines at individual scales can spur peer-to-peer engagement and catalyze the involvement of community leaders. One such example comes from Randolph County in rural southwest Georgia, which had been hit particularly hard by the pandemic. There, a nonpartisan vaccine initiative used door-to-door engagement—similar to conventional canvassing efforts—to reach individuals and explain the benefits of vaccination.[61] This model of engagement goes beyond a one-size-fits-all message delivered from a national authority and leverages trusted leaders and community members to work with and in the community they know best. Beyond getting the good word out, infrastructure investment should also prioritize increased access (i.e., bringing vaccines to where people are), an issue of particular importance for marginalized communities.

But access alone is not the only barrier.

The politicization of vaccines along partisan lines is disturbing. The increase in social media and influencer-driven sentiment against vaccination, spurred in part by discredited studies that link vaccination to autism, have set the backdrop for a predominantly Republican pushback against vaccination.[62] Some of the pushback derives from extreme conspiracy theories, but some of the resistance does have a semblance of logic—much of it framed around asymptomatic spread and the benefits of "natural immunity." First, if individuals often have asymptomatic cases, then the risk of infection is not nearly as great. Specifically, if there are side effects to a mRNA vaccine, then it would be ethical to balance those risks against the potential benefits, especially in groups where the relative risks of infection are low (like in healthy adolescents and young adults). Large-scale studies have found that the risk of severe outcomes (e.g., arrythmias or multi-inflammatory syndrome) in adolescents and healthy young adults who are infected outweighs the associated rare risks from vaccines.[63] Such evidence also indicates that the direct benefits of vaccination are lower for healthy adolescents and young adults. These grains of truth can become mountains of doubt in young adults, including women who are pregnant or breastfeeding.[64] Second, it is also likely that long-term protection is stronger from an infection than from a primary vaccination dose. But there is an enormous caveat. Such an outcome is conditional on surviving a SARS-CoV-2 infection, in which death is only the most extreme of many bad outcomes. By comparison, even though there may be rare adverse events associated with the vaccines,[65] the reality is that more than 1 million individuals have died of COVID-19 in the United States alone. At the population scale, there is no comparison between the two options. Although both infections and vaccines can increase population immunity, vaccination represents the safe and ethical way for both individuals and the population as a whole.

In moving forward, one of the central points of concern is that there is a false paradigm in place—namely, that "one is done." This concern applies to communities that have been willing to be vaccinated, communities that faced doubts but overcame them, and especially for communities that remain resistant to the idea of vaccination in the first place. The reality is that one is not done, and two is not even done. The initial two-dose series of vaccines showed more than a 90% decrease in hospitalization and fatalities when comparing those who were vaccinated with those who were not vaccinated. But the time course of the trial and the timing of the separation between doses was a balance between understanding the immune system and expediency. Ethical considerations required that comparisons be made between doses that involved relatively short time differences. Given the rate of infection and fatalities, there was not the luxury of waiting to learn if the ideal dosing schedule involved a three-dose series with a third dose administered many months after the initial doses. Striving for perfection comes with a cost. Instead, it became apparent that an initial two-dose series protects against severe illness, but it does not necessarily prevent asymptomatic infections (and transmission). Moreover, with time, the risk of both having an infection and having a severe illness increases. As a result, boosters have been needed, not only to deliver more of the same information on the shape of viral proteins in the original SARS-CoV-2 strain but potentially more of something different.

There is precedence and widespread acceptance of other types of boosters. The tetanus vaccine is one example. Tetanus is an awful disease. Also known as lockjaw, tetanus is caused by a bacteria *Clostridium tetani* that releases harmful endotoxins that can lead to muscle spasms, paralysis, and death in 20% of infections. There is no cure. But tetanus is easily preventable with timely administration of vaccines. First administered to children and then again as teens, adults should receive a tetanus booster (one known as Td, which covers tetanus and diphtheria, and one known as Tdap, which also covers pertussis) every 10 years.[66] These booster shots are widely accepted, are delivered as part of routine patient care, and are required for entry into the vast majority of colleges following recommendations from the American College Health Association.[67] Thankfully, the social norm in the United States remains in favor of routine vaccinations, some of which require repeated administration of boosters. Investment will be required to prepare us for repeated use of boosters against COVID-19—even if the question remains how best to do so.

Updating the content of mRNA vaccines to fight the viruses of today (and tomorrow)

In July 2021, a group of scientists shared a critically important line of evidence in the *New England Journal of Medicine*: boosters had a profound effect on the reduction of both confirmed COVID-19 infections and severe illness associated with hospitalization.[68] A comparison of outcomes among older individuals who had previously had a vaccine in early 2021 showed a more than 90% reduction in risk in the booster group relative to the group who had been vaccinated and not boosted. These boosters represented a repeat of the same mRNA vaccine provided earlier in the year. This early evidence was reinforced by public health decisions in the United States, Europe and elsewhere: the two-dose mRNA series was in fact a multidose series—a decision reflected in the recommendation that individuals receive a booster and then a second bivalent booster to benefit from maximal protection conferred from vaccines.[69] This evidence is key: boosters can protect individuals from infection and therefore reduce transmission chains that could lead to severe outcomes or worse.

Yet, we are not facing the same virus as before—the emergence of new variants has been rapid, sometimes unexpectedly so. Indeed, the same scientific group released a follow-up study in April 2022 showing that although a fourth mRNA vaccine dose provided some improvement over three doses, the effects were not nearly as striking as the relative impact of the booster compared to the original two-dose series.[70] Altogether, this suggests that preserving the efficacy of vaccination on a large scale requires scientific advances to update boosters to improve their effectiveness against present and future viruses and parallel efforts to sustain trust in the very mission of vaccinations at global scales.[71]

First, boosters. As already explained, the mRNA technology works by introducing a message at the injection site that our own cells use to generate the equivalent of viral debris—small bits and pieces that, in and of themselves, cannot make a functional virus. Instead, the debris is a signal to the immune system to learn to identify this foreign invader and prepare to fight back if it appears again. The target of the mRNA vaccines has been the "spike" protein—the semi-barbell-shaped macromolecule that gives SARS-CoV-2 its distinctive shape.[72] It is worthwhile to note that this target has long been suspected of having the right features, beginning with research on coronavirus vaccines in the wake of SARS-1. The spike protein is both essential for infection and elicits a strong immune response.[73] But the spike protein of the past is not necessarily the spike protein of today or tomorrow. As a result, if boosters continue to provide the same message, then it is possible that the immune system is preparing to fight the wrong enemy. The immune system will see an increase in a particular kind of spike protein and then increase the fraction of its immune repertoire dedicated to warding off that particular kind of virus. Instead, updating the mRNA vaccines requires that the pipeline of development becomes not a singular event but a process of continual improvement that combines real-time genomic monitoring with the production pipelines used to ensure that new mRNA messages are stable and likely to reflect the circulating viruses present when the vaccine is released. This process is followed by a series of trials meant to evaluate safety, efficacy, and efficacy at scale as part of critically timed updates. The process may end up resembling that of the influenza vaccine, or perhaps a "universal" SARS-CoV-2 vaccine will be developed.[74] Either way, updating boosters to protect the population should continue to have the goal of reducing the number of severe outcomes—specifically hospitalizations and fatalities.

Reaching this goal means that public health communications must be clearer regarding the purpose of boosters. If boosters protect against severe outcomes but less so against asymptomatic infections, or perhaps even turn a potentially symptomatic infection into an asymptomatic one, then this must be stated clearly. In light of evolution, a vaccine booster may not completely stop the risk of being infected, but it can reduce the risk of being severely harmed by an infection. This kind of communication can refocus individuals and the media back to the goal of vaccines: to take a disease that sometimes causes asymptomatic outcomes and sometimes causes severe outcomes to one that almost invariably causes an asymptomatic outcome. If that is the case, then the chain of harm is reduced, even if not entirely. If individuals who are vaccinated and boosted can get infected, then there may be shorter periods of inconvenience where they experience fatigue, headache, or fever, but they will be far less likely to experience the critical shortness of breath and low levels of oxygen delivery that put far too many people into hospitals, onto ventilators, and worse. Clarifying this goal will also help to reset expectations and defang some of the logic-adjacent based critiques (i.e., why get vaccinated if you can still get infected?). The point should be made clearly: when you are up to date on vaccines (as evaluation of boosters allows), then you may be infected, but you will have a much lower risk of severe infection, hospitalization, or death. Improving the communication of that message also requires that public health authorities understand which communities are most vulnerable—but that will require a different approach that goes beyond vaccination of individuals. Instead, new investment is needed to understand the breakdown of prior infections, vaccinations, and how the accumulation of these exposures changes the likelihood of severe outcomes as case levels change and as the virus evolves.

Developing a framework for population-wide immune surveys and future vulnerability

The start of this book explored the scientific basis for one of the earliest debates surrounding the impact of COVID-19: how many people had actually been infected. It was apparent that many more individuals were being infected than those documented in case reports alone. But precisely how many became controversial because of a dearth in testing—that then led to an opportunity for some to claim that perhaps 100-fold as many infections had occurred for each documented case. If true, COVID-19 should have flamed out in spring or summer 2020—but it did not. Instead, the use of serological surveys began to fill in the gaps, showing that there were approximately 6 to 24 times the number of actual infections for each documented case in the early stage of the pandemic[75] and approximately 4 to 5 times the number of actual infections for each documented case cumulatively through 2020.[76]

But there are many other reasons to use serological surveys.[77] For example, before the development of vaccines, individuals who had recovered from infections and were therefore significantly less likely to experience another near-term infection could have been part of shield immunity strategies—that is, increasing their interactions with potentially vulnerable individuals and reducing the risk that asymptomatically infected individuals passed on infections to susceptible individuals.[78,79,80] Indeed, the use of health passes in Europe are an example of a variation on this theme that emerged only after the introduction of vaccines. Serological surveys could have another role, too—they could provide a reflection of the ways in which the ebb and flow of immunity is shaped by prior infections, vaccinations, and changes in the virus itself.

This chapter already introduced the concept of population immunity in terms of the fraction of individuals in a focal population who are no longer immunologically naive to SARS-CoV-2. This aggregate index can increase in one of two ways: through vaccinations and through infections. Yet, if we think about an effective interpretation, then the exposure to SARS-CoV-2 in February 2021 may mean something very different from an exposure in the past month—the same holds true for receiving the initial two dose mRNA vaccine series versus receiving a recent booster. Even if one is no longer immunologically naive, one can still become increasingly immunologically vulnerable. Hence, the timing of waves and vaccination campaigns structure population-level protection; linking the two and understanding the durability of vaccination-based and infection-based immunity requires a new investment that views immunity as heterogeneous and dynamic.

There are opportunities. The CDC already has a surveillance infrastructure in place that could be leveraged to examine who has antibodies, how many people have recently been infected, and what variants were present during each wave.[81] This infrastructure comes with biases, given the link between access to health care and the likelihood of being included in a serosurvey. Nonetheless, linking this serosurvey information to hospital admissions and fatalities can explain at the population scale precisely why individuals (and which individuals) should seek a booster. Public health authorities might even go one step further, developing cohorts that are followed with time, similar to other large cohort studies, in which outcomes are linked to individualized choices on vaccines as well as sufficiently regular viral testing to connect infections, vaccines, and outcomes. These two types of studies—snapshot and longitudinal—would provide complementary information to inform decision-making. Thus far, the evidence has remained strong that vaccines are the most effective and ethical approach to reduce the risk of a severe infection. But, there is no guarantee that this message will be durable in the face of evolving variants. And, if the old set of vaccines are no longer effective, then both the message and vaccines must be updated.

In doing so, one key message must also shine through: we are connected, and the most immunologically vulnerable parts of the United States and the world will inevitably become the gateway for more spread, more evolution, and a rebound back into locations that thought that they had COVID-19 under control. There have been many studies that have pointed out the ethical flaws of a vaccination policy that centers on the United States (or other developed countries) alone.[82,83,84] Such ethical arguments are important. But, they do not appeal to all. If vaccines are limited, what is the benefit of vaccinating others? Why not use these vaccines to protect our own population?

There is in fact a different kind of answer to this question, one that starts from the selfish perspective and ends up in an altruistic frame. The premise is simple. If vaccines are available in a rich nation, should the rich nation donate part of its supply to a less-well-off but connected neighboring nation, even if the rich nation has a selfish objective in mind: to reduce the number of its fatalities. At face value, it would seem that the optimal approach would be to not share. It turns out that this is wrong. When vaccine distribution is relatively slow—a hallmark of the US response—then sharing part of a vaccine stockpile with neighbor nations has a secondary benefit: it reduces the intensity of outbreaks elsewhere, which in turn reduces the intensity of new infections introduced through travel between nations.[85] As a result, sharing can be beneficial—in a purely selfish sense—thereby improving the public health landscape both locally and globally. This argument of reaching an ethical endpoint through a purely selfish objective also contains a lesson. We live in a connected world, and if we only think about problems in the United States, we are bound to fight a far worse fight than if we were to fight the war against emerging infectious diseases with allies around the world.

The preceding sections focused on steps to build a resilient population immunity and make it more likely that infections are mild or asymptomatic—not just for individuals but for the population as a whole. If implemented thoughtfully, at scale, and inclusively with the participation of the population they serve, we may be able to move toward a situation where mild or asymptomatic COVID-19 infections become the norm. Eventually—as was the case in 2023—then total fatalities will start to decrease further and further. This is the near-term promise of COVID-19 vaccines—not to stop all infections but to make a dramatic difference in harm, both for individuals and the population. While part 1 ended with the finding that asymptomatic infections can increase total fatalities, the story of vaccines may be one in which making mild or asymptomatic outcomes the norm can systematically drive down fatalities for populations as a whole.

In closing, mRNA vaccine technology is a wonderful development, but it comes with limits. The United States is large, heterogeneous, and increasingly divided. We do not necessarily agree on the need for vaccines to fight a virus that killed more than 1 million Americans in a little over two years. The impact of any technological advancement will be limited if we do not also engage with individuals, their social networks, and community leaders and find more than one way to talk about the potential for vaccines to save lives and loved ones. These conversations represent as monumental a task—perhaps even more so—than the science that has made the conversation possible.

Coda

Infrastructure Investment for a Better Normal

COVID-19 is not going away.

Instead, COVID-19 will continue to spread from human to human, replicate, mutate, generate new variants, and challenge our ability to return to "normal." On the other hand, we—as individuals or as societies—may decide that we have moved on, putting aside our masks (even when visiting nursing homes), returning to large events, opting not to test, neglecting the use of vaccines, and accepting the status quo with respect to the quality of air we breathe. If we do that—or accept that from business and school leaders and from elected officials spanning cities, counties, states, and the federal government—then we will have missed our chance to genuinely return to a better normal.

A better normal would be one in which we change our policies and use new technology to transform the environmental preconditions and social norms that made COVID-19 so devastating, given the viral mechanism of asymptomatic spread that allows it to evade conventional efforts of containment. Reaching a better normal that can improve baseline health and reduce the risk of pandemics will not be easy—good things usually take hard work. But in the absence of hard work, we are setting ourselves up for a worse future.

As this book already showed, many individuals, groups, and a few nongovernmental institutions reacted rapidly to the pandemic threat and took hard steps to fight back in productive, science-driven, and compassionate ways. With the right investment, these grassroots efforts could be combined with corporate-governmental vaccine initiatives to form the basis for a sustainable pandemic control and prevention infrastructure at the local and national levels.

What would the end result look like?

Each one of us should be able to walk into indoor spaces and expect not to breathe in a steady stream of respiratory viruses floating in unfiltered air. In other words, any sustainable approach to deal with future respiratory disease pandemics must confront the problem of asymptomatic transmission that can turn an innocuous indoor gathering into a superspreading event. If this is to happen, we need to do more than generate reactive responses wave after wave. We need sustainable approaches to prevent spread, especially when few people are sick and there is an opportunity to halt transmission at early stages. In essence, we need a pandemic infrastructure that prioritizes prevention, not just control, because a rapidly spreading outbreak is far harder (and more expensive) to control, and it may not be controllable at all.

Transforming infrastructure is a hard problem to solve—and the United States remains far from achieving the kind of core support that we like to imagine represents a baseline for functional countries— particularly those as rich as the United States is, at least when measured in terms of gross domestic product.

In functional nations, it should be possible to send your children to a public school that gives them a high-quality civic and technical education.

In functional nations, it should be possible to drink lead-free and pesticide-free water from the kitchen tap and even in water fountains in public squares.

In functional nations, it should be possible to go for walks in city parks or forests and breath in fresh air—and not a toxic mix of smog and pollutants.

Many of America's cities and states do not meet these standards, a problem not confined to Flint, Michigan,[1] or Jackson, Mississippi,[2] or East Palestine, Ohio.[3] There are many hurdles to fixing public schools, water quality, air quality, bridges, and roads. These are thorny problems that are compounded and in some cases driven by long-standing inequities such that a good school, clean water, or a fresh breeze is "something for me and not for thee." These inequities make it harder, if not impossible, for children in Flint, Appalachia, or El Paso, and far too many other children across the United States, to get a fair shot.

Likewise, if we are to make sustainable progress in confronting COVID-19 and infectious diseases more generally, then we have to fix the pathways in which one case becomes many. If we do so in the right way, then people from all walks of life who must balance work, family, social obligations, and stresses do not need to become pandemic experts. Instead, expertise should be leveraged to transform built environments, making it possible to improve health and socioeconomic outcomes jointly, without blaming the very people hurt (sometimes irrevocably) by institutional and societal failures in preparing for a global pandemic.

In early 2022, a multidisciplinary group of more than 20 scientists, physicians, engineers, business leaders, and policymakers issued a pandemic response roadmap report that identifies more than a dozen priority areas for action-taking to prevent future pandemics.[4] These recommendations span testing, vaccines, air quality, therapeutics, communication, workforce development, and beyond. These are precisely the kinds of recommendations necessary to drive national-level policy and investment. But in doing so, we should not lose sight of overarching themes that underlie specific policy recommendations. That is, if we do not explain the central epidemiological lessons of how COVID-19 spread, who it hurts the most, and how we can short-circuit asymptomatic pathways, then we will lose the opportunity to help many understand, support, and engage with public health campaigns and investment.

The first part of this book developed a generalized argument for why COVID-19 was so devastating, centering on a simple but paradoxical premise. Asymptomatic infections may be good news for an individual but bad news for populations. The mix of asymptomatic and symptomatic transmission means that asymptomatic infections can silently enable a virus to reach vulnerable individuals and increase the total number of severe cases and fatalities when compared to similar diseases where transmission is linked to symptoms. The reality of mild and asymptomatic cases also catalyzed a plausible counternarrative: that the disease was, in effect, harmless or at least no worse than seasonal flu. This counternarrative was flawed from the start. The false notion that COVID-19 was no worse than seasonal flu is a key reason why it has been necessary to launch a joint campaign: both against the virus and against flawed narratives. Combating future pandemics requires that we evaluate evidence for asymptomatic spread and then explain why stopping mild or asymptomatic cases is precisely the mechanism needed to prevent serious infections, hospitalizations, and deaths for the population as a whole.

The second part of this book responded to this central premise by identifying three major approaches to fight back against asymptomatic infection and transmission. These approaches addressed perception gaps and translated scientific principles into practical opportunities to reduce transmission and the severity of infection. The chapters covered the science and deployment of (i) risk communication platforms that link data gathering to localized, real-time assessments connected to events most likely to catalyze new cases—while working to reduce risk in indoor environments through clear indoor air initiatives; (ii) large-scale viral testing programs meant to identify and isolate asymptomatic individuals before they have a chance to infect others; (iii) large-scale vaccination campaigns to reduce severe disease and fatalities. These are only some of the ways in which providing a core rationale for action-taking can strengthen the case for infrastructure development in the first place and help persuade individuals to take actions when individualized responses are needed.

The chain of asymptomatic transmission starts with an infectious individual—someone who feels fine but is nonetheless shedding infectious virus particles indoors, without a mask, in a poorly ventilated space. This one sentence points out ways in which asymptomatic transmission becomes the mechanism to motivate change. The chance that an individual is infected is fundamentally related to the state of the pandemic—that is, how many people are infected at a given time.

The difficulty of finding asymptomatic infections means, however, that we are invariably faced with case data that both lags in time and is significantly underreported. Next, when a person enters into a space, then the chances that they infect others depends on whether the indoor space is in fact sufficiently well ventilated and equipped with air filters that can reduce the density of potentially infectious particles in the air. Such ventilation and filtering are far from the norm.

Of course, there may be circumstances where the combination of high densities of individuals and filtering capacity means that there is no safe guarantee of a low-risk air environment. In those cases—whether because of the nature of the space (e.g., crowded buses, trains, and planes) and/or the nature of the people in the facility (e.g., nursing homes and other long-term care facilities)—it will be key to view indoor space as heterogeneous and not resort to a one-size-fits-all solution to interventions, including mask-wearing. Tiered systems will be required to treat airborne risk levels differently in different circumstances.

Finally, even if one is exposed and infected, what happens next also depends on how much we have done in advance, especially with respect to vaccinating the most vulnerable—including those who are at highest risk of severe outcomes (e.g., the elderly, the immunocompromised, the very young, and those unable to receive the vaccine). For COVID-19, the evidence of a J-shaped risk curve meant that the elderly were significantly more likely to have a severe infection, be hospitalized, or die than any other age group. Future pandemics may have other characteristic risk shapes. Large-scale vaccination campaigns can be made more compelling if we recognize that the mix of vaccine-derived and infection-derived immunity transforms both the epidemic rates of spread as well as the threat of a severe outcome to an individual. It also requires that we communicate the protective value of vaccines while being frank about the different risks that come with age and different histories of interactions with the virus and vaccines.

COVID-19's J-shaped curve means there is a relatively low risk of hospitalization and fatality for children and young adults and a relatively high risk of hospitalization and fatality for the elderly. This fact offers little consolation to those who lost loved ones of any age. Nonetheless, it could have been different and even worse. COVID-19's severity could have followed a U-shape curve in which there is a high risk of severe outcomes for both the young and old.[5] Even healthy young adults can be at risk from other infectious diseases. Consider pertussis, which disproportionately causes severe outcomes in infants under six months and children who have not yet completed their vaccinations (as well as the elderly),[6] and the 1918 pandemic influenza H1N1 strain, which killed 50 million people worldwide (with elevated mortality rates in children, young adults, and the elderly).[7]

We can hope to remain "lucky" in the future such that risk to the young remains low even as the virus evolves—but hope is not enough. We must continue to be vigilant and focus on the development and evaluation of vaccines for all ages while recognizing that up-to-date data is required to prioritize vaccines for those most likely to have severe cases, especially as viruses evolve and immunity wanes in an individual's lifetime.

This multilayered arc of intervention starts with a premise: asymptomatic transmission has been and will remain a double-edge sword. But, if we can transform the state of our indoor spaces, systematically address gaps in immunity, and use targeted data-driven approaches to let individuals leverage public health resources to protect their own health, then perhaps we may finally move COVID-19 into a new category: a disease that predominantly causes asymptomatic or mild cases without the double edge.

If there is one lesson in this book, it is this: by facing why we failed to stop COVID-19 from becoming a societally transforming event, we may be able to develop sustainable approaches to build a better normal. In doing so, we will have a chance to control the spread of COVID-19 in the near term and help prevent the spread of pandemics to come.

ACKNOWLEDGMENTS

In January 2022, after two intensive years spent working on COVID-19 modeling and response, I decided to step back from the daily cycle to synthesize and communicate a broader view. The first draft of this book was written in spring 2022 while I was on a faculty development leave from Georgia Tech. The final version reflects the input and advice of many whose critique improved the text immeasurably. There is a long list of friends, colleagues, and collaborators to thank, all of whom helped improve my understanding of what we were up against and what could be done to make a meaningful difference. Together, I hope our collaborative research and interventions have made an impact in helping individuals and public health decision-makers fight back against a formidable pathogen. Any remaining mistakes or lack of clarity in the text are my fault alone.

I am grateful to the many students and early career researchers in my Quantitative Viral Dynamics group who went above and beyond to respond in a time-sensitive fashion to new information and demands for yet another model, plot, or analysis. I offer my thanks to many close collaborators for their contributions and input, including Stephen Beckett, Freyja A. Brandel-Tanis, Aroon Chande, Caitlin Cheung, Ashley Coenen, David Demory, Marian Dominguez-Mirazo, Esther Gallmeier, Jeremy Harris, Seolha Lee, Joey Leung, Guanlin Li, Andreea Magalie, Daniel Muratore, Quan Nguyen, Rogelio Rodriguez-Gonzalez, Adriana Lucia Sanz, Shashwat Shivam, and Conan Zhao.

In addition, I am grateful to all those colleagues at Georgia Tech who worked to develop, deploy, support, and manage the campus asymptomatic testing initiative from summer 2020 to summer 2022—particularly Greg Gibson, Michael Shannon, Benjamin Holton, Anton Bryksin, Brian Liu, Madeline Sieglinger, Renee Kopkowski, Sandi

Bramblett, JulieAnne Williamson, Michael Farrell, Alexander Ortiz, Chaouki Abdallah, Andrés García, and Frank Neville. This list is only partial, as the success of our intervention effort would not have been possible without the support of students, staff, and faculty of the campus community, as well as the institute leadership and support of President Ángel Cabrera.

Likewise, I am grateful to the many colleagues who codeveloped our COVID-19 Event Risk Assessment Planning Tool, supported our communication efforts, and have made it possible to evaluate its impact over multiple years, with special thanks and acknowledgments to the contributions of Aroon Chande, Troy Hilley, Lavanya Rishishwar, Stephen Beckett, Freyja A. Brandel-Tanis, Audra Davidson, Jess Hunt-Ralston, Allie Sinclair, Morgan Taylor, Alison Adcock, Greg Samanez-Larkin, and Clio Andris.

Beyond my institutional colleagues, I am grateful to have worked with so many talented collaborators and colleagues in COVID-19 modeling and response efforts, including Carly Adams, Avnika Amin, Henri Berestycki, Ben Bolker, David Champredon, Matthew Collins, Daniel Cornforth, Giulia de Meijere, Benoit Desjardins, David Earn, Ceyhun Eksin, Scott Fridkin, Sebastian Funk, C. Franklin Goldsmith, Bryan Grenfell, Michael Hochberg, Joseph Kellogg, Alicia Kraay, Michael Li, Andrew Medford, Jessica Metcalf, Martial Ndeffo, Kristin Nelson, Jean-Marc Oury, Andrew Peterson, Christopher Rose, Aaron Siegler, Kayoko Shioda, Patrick Sullivan, Tejs Vegge, and Yorai Wardi, These collaborations would not have been possible without the support of two outstanding scientists who transitioned into critical roles as project coordinators—Jessica Irons and Gabi Steinbach.

The perspective of this book was shaped by the support of many funding agencies and their program officers who recognized and graciously gave our team the green light to respond in a time of national need. The research and communication efforts were made possible by support from the National Science Foundation's programs in Envirommental Biology, the Physics of Living Systems, Bridging Ecology and Evolution, Ecology of Infectious Disease, Biological Oceanography, and Computing and Communication Foundations; the National

Institutes of Health's National Institute of Allergy and Infectious Diseases and National Institute of General Medical Sciences; and the Simons Foundation, Army Research Office, Burroughs Wellcome Fund, Centers for Disease Control and Prevention, Rockefeller Foundation, Charities in Aid Foundation, the Marier Cunningham Foundation, Clark Foundation, and the Île-de-France region.

My perspective on how to respond to COVID-19 has been shaped by new and old friends and colleagues. I am deeply grateful to Jonathan Dushoff, Sang Woo Park, and Benjamin Lopman for responding to more daytime and late-night queries than I can count. Their insight into how epidemics unfold and what we as individuals and as societies can do to control them has been deeply influential to my synthesis. I am also grateful to the input of two anonymous reviewers and three additional careful readers, Audra Davidson, Mallory Harris, and Benjamin Lopman (yet again), whose eye for science and accessibility greatly improved the text.

I am also thankful for the many discussions and exchanges on what COVID-19 could become and what it meant outside the ivory tower, with particular thanks to Shweta Bansal, Trevor Bedford, Ana Bento, Carl Bergstrom, Ian Bogost, Maïa Brami, Vittoria Colizza, Ofer Cornfeld, Dan Cunningham, Florence Débarre, Carlos del Rio, Rachel Dempsey, Joy Depenbrok, Otto Depenbrok, Michael Desai, Steve Diggle, Peter Dodds, Chris Dolan, Jeremy Faust, Michael Fischer, Spencer Fox, Nigel Goldenfeld, Daniel Goldman, Michael Goodisman, Abba Gumel, Chen Halevi, Pinar Keskinocak, Julia Kubanek, Daniel Larremore, Rich Lenski, Marc Lipsitch, Neysun Mahboubi, Troy McKenzie, Lauren Meyers, Janet Murray, Richard Neher, B. Aditya Prakash, Sam Scarpino, Amber Schmidtke, Rachel Slayton, Todd Streelman, Eran Yashiv, and Andrew Zangwill. I am also grateful to Bill Nigut for his kind series of invitations to join him and guests on Georgia Public Broadcasting to explain the threat posed by COVID-19; his insightful questions that spanned public health to politics were critical in shaping how I prioritized my time and communicated our ongoing research findings.

Thank you to Joe Rusko and Suzanne Staszak-Silva at Johns Hopkins University Press, who saw the potential for this book to reach a broader audience and to the team of editors and production specialists for making this project possible.

Finally, my deepest thanks to Maira, Ilan, and Noa for supporting me even as I worked endlessly on what seemed like an endless pandemic. I am hopeful that this book can help inform the type of science-driven investment and action-taking that leads to meaningful change.

antigen test: A rapid assay that returns a positive when an individual is shedding viral particles that contain small molecular signatures that can bind against a predefined antibody. In practice, the tests can return results in 15 minutes, similar to rapid pregnancy tests. A true-positive test means that an individual is shedding virus (and is likely infectious).

average duration of infectiousness: The average period of time during which an individual infects other individuals, as averaged across individuals in a population. For SARS-CoV-2, individuals may have varying levels of infectious virus in their lungs and upper nasal passageways, such that varying levels of infectious virus are released in the air when they exhale. Near the start and end of the infectious period, their viral load will be low enough that it would likely take extended interaction in a poorly ventilated indoor space for a susceptible person who is exposed to become infected. Whereas, near the peak of their infectious period, it is possible that even an incidental close interaction without a mask could lead to an infection in a susceptible person

case fatality rate (CFR): The number of documented fatalities divided by the number of documented cases. Both the numerator (fatalities) and denominator (cases) may be underestimates.

Ct value: The "cycle threshold" value (abbreviated as Ct) represents the number of doubling cycles required to detect a viral signal in a PCR test (see Glossary for definition of PCR test).

epidemic speed: The exponential rate at which cases double over time.

epidemic strength. *See* reproduction number (basic) and reproduction number (effective).

final size: The fraction of individuals in a population infected when an epidemic comes to an end (can also be applied to estimate the fraction of individuals infected by a particular variant).

herd immunity: A state in which a critical fraction of a population has either been vaccinated or has recovered from a disease and is presumed to be (temporarily) immune from near-term infection, at which point the number of new cases is expected to go down with time.

incidence: The number of new cases per time, such as the number of new cases per day or week.

infection fatality rate (IFR): The number of fatalities divided by the number of actual infections.

PCR (polymerase chain reaction) test: A molecular viral test that evaluates whether or not an individual has the genetic material of a focal virus. A positive PCR test result does not necessarily imply the individual is infectious. A true-positive test means that the individual was recently exposed (and will soon be infectious), are currently infectious, or have recovered (and are not infectious) but still shedding noninfectious viral remnants. PCR tests usually take 24 hours to return an answer, but same-day turnaround times are possible.

reproduction number (basic): The average number of new infections caused by a single infectious individual in an otherwise susceptible (local) population, denoted as R_0. When this number is less than one, an infection is less likely to spread in a new population.

reproduction number (effective): The average number of new infections caused by a single infectious individual in a partially susceptible (local) population, denoted as R_{eff}. When this number is less than one, the rate of new cases is expected to decrease.

SARS-CoV-2: An RNA virus from the coronavirus family. Individual virus particles consist of a positive-sense, single-stranded RNA genome encapsulated by a nucleocapsid protein, which itself is surrounded by a membrane and a structural protein envelope. Spike proteins protrude from the envelope and enable recognition and binding to human cells and the initiation of infection.

sensitivity and specificity: These are two measures of medical test statistics: sensitivity is the extent to which an individual who is actually positive for the condition (i.e., is infected) returns a positive test result; specificity is the extent to which an individual who is negative for the condition (i.e., is not infected) returns a negative result.

serial interval: The time between when an infector exhibits symptoms and the time the person they infect (the infectee) exhibits symptoms. The serial interval is typically positive (i.e., a few days in the case of COVID-19), but it can be zero or even negative, such as when a presymptomatic individual infects someone else who then exhibits symptoms earlier than the person who infected them.

serological test (or antibody test): A test that takes serum from blood and evaluates it for the presence of antibodies against a particular pathogen. The antibodies specifically bind against a panel of targeted antigens. A positive test means that the individual has recently been infected. A negative test could mean that the individual was not recently infected, was recently infected but has not yet developed sufficient levels of antibodies, or was infected a longer time ago and the antibodies dropped below detectable levels.

vaccination threshold: The vaccination threshold refers to the levels of vaccination in a focal population that would imply that the basic reproduction number is below one. As a result, a random vaccination campaign that has exceeded the vaccination threshold should be able to contain the emergence of outbreaks in the population at large, although clusters of unvaccinated communities could still experience outbreaks.

Chapter 1. It Was Never Just "the Flu"

1. Azad, A. (2020, April 13). An influential model projects coronavirus deaths will stop this summer, but experts are skeptical. CNN. https://www.cnn.com/2020/04/13/health/ihme-model-death-predictions/index.html.

2. Moreland, A., et al. (2020). Timing of state and territorial COVID-19 stay-at-home orders and changes in population movement—United States, March 1–May 31, 2020. *MMWR* 69: 1198–1203. https://doi.org/10.15585/mmwr.mm6935a2.

3. Gates Foundation. (2017, January 25). Bill & Melinda Gates Foundation boosts vital work of the University of Washington's Institute for Health Metrics and Evaluation (news release). https://www.gatesfoundation.org/ideas/media-center/press-releases/2017/01/ihme-announcement.

4. Staffing figures are from the IHME website (https://www.healthdata.org/).

5. See note 1.

6. See note 1.

7. See note 1.

8. Jewell, N.P., Lewnard, J.A., and Jewell, B.L. (2020). Caution warranted: Using the Institute for Health Metrics and Evaluation model for predicting the course of the COVID-19 pandemic. *Annals of Internal Medicine* 173: 226–227. https://doi.org/10.7326/M20-1565.

9. The COVID Tracking Project. (n.d.). The Atlantic Monthly Group. https://covidtracking.com/data/national.

10. Russell, T.W., et al. (2020). Estimating the infection and case fatality ratio for coronavirus disease (COVID-19) using age-adjusted data from the outbreak on the Diamond Princess cruise ship, February 2020. *Eurosurveillance* 25: 2000256. https://doi.org/10.2807/1560-7917.ES.2020.25.12.2000256.

11. See note 9.

12. Havers F.P., et al. (2020). Seroprevalence of antibodies to SARS-CoV-2 in 10 sites in the United States, March 23–May 12, 2020. *JAMA Internal Medicine* 180: 1576–1586. https://doi.org/10.1001/jamainternmed.2020.4130.

13. Back, A.L., Arnold, R.M., and Quill, T.E. (2003). Hope for the best, and prepare for the worst. *Annals of Internal Medicine* 138: 439–443. https://doi.org/10.7326/0003-4819-138-5-200303040-00028.

14. Error function. (n.d.). Wikipedia. https://en.wikipedia.org/wiki/Error_function.

15. Farr, W. (1839). *Progress of Epidemics—Epidemic of Small Pox in Annual Report of the Registrar-General of Births, Deaths, and Marriages in England*. HMSO, London. https://babel.hathitrust.org/cgi/pt?id=njp.32101064041955&view=1up&seq=89.

16. De Kruif, P. (2002). *Microbe Hunters*. Harcourt, San Diego, CA. Originally published in 1926.

17. Van Helvoort, T., and Sankaran, N. (2019). How seeing became knowing: The role of the electron microscope in shaping the modern definition of viruses. *Journal of the History of Biology* 52: 125–160.

18. Bregman, D.J., and Langmuir, A.D. (1990). Farr's law applied to AIDS projections. *JAMA* 263: 1522–1525. https://doi.org/10.1001/jama.1990.03440110088033.

19. See note 18.

20. First 500,000 AIDS cases—United States. (1995, November 24). *MMWR* 44: 849–853.

21. World Health Organization. (n.d.). Data on the size of the HIV epidemic. https://www.who.int/data/gho/data/themes/topics/topic-details/GHO/data-on-the-size-of-the-hiv-aids-epidemic.

22. Silver, N. (2020, April 17). Tweet. https://twitter.com/NateSilver538/status/1251143348536127488?s=20&t=IxMAze5rvUptPVJRTYfLRQ.

23. Tankersly, J. (2020, May 6). No virus deaths by mid-May? White House economists say they didn't forecast early end to fatalities. *New York Times*. https://www.nytimes.com/2020/05/06/business/coronavirus-white-house-economists.html.

24. Council of Economic Advisers 45 (CEA45) Archived. (2020, May 5). Tweet. https://twitter.com/WhiteHouseCEA45/status/1257680258364555264.

25. Azzoni, T., and Dampf, A. (2020, May 25). Game zero: Spread of virus linked to Champions League match. Associated Press. https://apnews.com/article/milan-la-liga-ap-top-news-valencia-virus-outbreak-ae59cfc0641fc63afd09182bb832ebe2.

26. Goodman, P.S., and Pianigiani G. (2020, November 19). Why Covid caused such suffering in Italy's wealthiest region. *New York Times*. https://www.nytimes.com/2020/11/19/business/lombardy-italy-coronavirus-doctors.html.

27. Cereda, D., et al. (2021). The early phase of the COVID-19 epidemic in Lombardy, Italy. *Epidemics* 37: 100528. https://doi.org/10.1016/j.epidem.2021.100528.

28. Ioannidis, J.P.A. (2020, March 17). A fiasco in the making? As the coronavirus pandemic takes hold, we are making decisions without reliable data. Stat. https://www.statnews.com/2020/03/17/a-fiasco-in-the-making-as-the-coronavirus-pandemic-takes-hold-we-are-making-decisions-without-reliable-data/.

29. Folkenflik, D. (2015, November 4). "Boston Globe" owner launches "Stat News" site covering life sciences. NPR. https://www.npr.org/2015/11/04/454692304/boston-globe-owner-launches-stat-news-site-covering-life-sciences.

30. See note 28.

31. Mizumoto, K., et al. (2020). Estimating the asymptomatic proportion of coronavirus disease 2019 (COVID-19) cases on board the Diamond Princess cruise ship, Yokohama, Japan, 2020. *Eurosurveillance* 25: 2000180. https://doi.org/10.2807/1560-7917.ES.2020.25.10.2000180.

32. See note 10.

33. See note 10.

34. See note 28.

35. US House Archives—Select Subcommittee on the Coronavirus Crisis (2022, June). The Atlas Dogma. https://coronavirus-democrats-oversight.house.gov/sites/democrats.coronavirus.house.gov/files/2022.06.21%20The%20Trump%20

Administration%E2%80%99s%20Embrace%20of%20a%20Dangerous%20and%20
Discredited%20Herd%20Immunity%20via%20Mass%20Infection%20Strategy.pdf.

36. Johns Hopkins Coronavirus Resource Center. (2022, May 17). U.S. officially
surpasses 1 million Covid-19 deaths. https://coronavirus.jhu.edu/from-our
-experts/u-s-officially-surpasses-1-million-covid-19-deaths.

37. Shuster, S. (2020, March 31). "I still can't believe what I'm seeing": What it's like
to live across the street from a temporary morgue during the coronavirus
outbreak. *Time*. https://time.com/5812569/covid-19-new-york-morgues/.

38. Feuer, A., and Salcedo, A. (2020, April 2). New York City deploys 45 mobile
morgues as virus strains funeral homes. *New York Times*. https://www.nytimes
.com/2020/04/02/nyregion/coronavirus-new-york-bodies.html.

39. Giuffrida, A. (2020, May 29). Why was Lombardy hit harder than Italy's other
regions? *The Guardian*. https://www.theguardian.com/world/2020/may/29/why
-was-lombardy-hit-harder-covid-19-than-italys-other-regions.

40. Johns Hopkins University Coronavirus Resource Center. (n.d.). Data timeline.
https://coronavirus.jhu.edu/region/us/new-york.

41. See note 28.

42. CDC. (2021, updated March 19). COVID-19 pandemic planning scenarios.
https://www.cdc.gov/coronavirus/2019-ncov/hcp/planning-scenarios.html.

43. Jackson, C.B., et al. (2022). Mechanisms of SARS-CoV-2 entry into cells. *Nature
Reviews Molecular Cell Biology* 23: 3–20. https://doi.org/10.1038/s41580-021-00418-x.

44. Judson, J.F. (1979). *The Eighth Day of Creation: The Makers of the Revolution in
Biology*. Simon & Schuster, New York.

45. Mina, M., Parker, R., and Larremore, D.B. (2020). Rethinking Covid-19 test
sensitivity—a strategy for containment. *New England Journal of Medicine* 383:
e120. https://doi.org/10.1056/NEJMp2025631.

46. Pisanic, N., et al. (2020). COVID-19 serology at population scale: SARS-CoV-2-
specific antibody responses in saliva. *Journal of Clinical Microbiology* 59: e02204-
20. https://doi.org/10.1128/JCM.02204-20.

47. Vogel, G. (2020, April 21). Antibody surveys suggesting vast undercount of
coronavirus infections may be unreliable: Critics question accuracy of tests and
media promotion before full results are published. *Science*. https://doi.org/10.1126
/science.abc3831.

48. Bendavid, E., et al. (2020). COVID-19 antibody seroprevalence in Santa Clara
County, California. MedRxiv. https://doi.org/10.1101/2020.04.14.20062463. See
the published version (2021) in *International Journal of Epidemiology* 50: 410–419.
https://doi.org/10.1093/ije/dyab010.

49. US House Archives—Select Subcommittee on the Coronavirus Crisis (2022,
June). The Atlas Dogma. https://coronavirus-democrats-oversight.house.gov/sites
/democrats.coronavirus.house.gov/files/2022.06.21%20The%20Trump%20
Administration%E2%80%99s%20Embrace%20of%20a%20Dangerous%20and%20
Discredited%20Herd%20Immunity%20via%20Mass%20Infection%20Strategy.pdf,

50. Dr. John Ioannidis testimony to US Senate. (2020, May 6). US Senate Committee
on Homeland Security and Governmental Affairs. https://www.hsgac.senate.gov
/imo/media/doc/Testimony-Ioannidis-2020-05-06.pdf.

51. Ioannidis, J. (2005). Why most published research findings are false. *PLOS Medicine* 2: e124. https://doi.org/10.1371/journal.pmed.0020124.

52. Mallapaty, S. (2020, April 17). Antibody tests suggest that coronavirus infections vastly exceed official counts. *Nature.* Article was updated on April 19 with comments from Marm Kilpatrick and corrected on April 22 with a new estimate of the false positive rate. https://www.nature.com/articles/d41586-020-01095-0.

53. See note 52.

54. Petersen, E., et al. (2020). Comparing SARS-CoV-2 with SARS-CoV and influenza pandemics. *The Lancet Infectious Diseases* 20: e238–e244. https://doi.org/10.1016/S1473-3099(20)30484-9.

55. Faust, J.S., and del Rio, C. (2020). Assessment of deaths from COVID-19 and from seasonal influenza. *JAMA Internal Medicine* 180: 1045–1046. https://doi.org/10.1001/jamainternmed.2020.2306.

56. CDC. (n.d.). About the underlying cause of death, 1999–2020. https://wonder.cdc.gov/ucd-icd10.html.

57. CDC. (2023, September 12 last reviewed). Excess deaths associated with COVID-19. https://www.cdc.gov/nchs/nvss/vsrr/covid19/excess_deaths.htm.

58. Woolf, S.W., et al. (2021). Excess deaths from COVID-19 and other causes in the US, March 1, 2020, to January 2, 2021. *JAMA* 325: 1786–1789. https://doi.org/10.1001/jama.2021.5199.

59. This statistic is from Johns Hopkins University Coronavirus Resource Center (https://coronavirus.jhu.edu/).

60. World Health Organization. (2021, May 20). The true death toll of COVID-19: Estimating global excess mortality. https://www.who.int/data/stories/the-true-death-toll-of-covid-19-estimating-global-excess-mortality.

61. Wang, H., et al. (2022). Estimating excess mortality due to the COVID-19 pandemic: A systematic analysis of COVID-19-related mortality, 2020–21. *The Lancet* 399: 1513–1536. https://doi.org/10.1016/S0140-6736(21)02796-3.

62. Glanz, J., Hvistendahl, M., and Chang, A. (2023, February 15). How deadly was China's Covid wave? *New York Times.* https://www.nytimes.com/interactive/2023/02/15/world/asia/china-covid-death-estimates.html.

63. Hawkins, R.B., Charles, E.J., and Mehaffey, J.H. (2020). Socio-economic status and COVID-19-related cases and fatalities. *Public Health* 189: 129–134. https://doi.org/10.1016/j.puhe.2020.09.016.

64. Hillis, S., et al. (2022). Orphanhood and caregiver loss among children based on new global excess COVID-19 death estimates. *JAMA Pediatrics* 176: 1145–1148. https://doi.org/10.1001/jamapediatrics.2022.3157.

Chapter 2. Mild Cases and Experiential Bubbles

1. Park, J.H., et al. (2010). Perceptions and behaviors related to hand hygiene for the prevention of H1N1 influenza transmission among Korean university students during the peak pandemic period. *BMC Infectious Diseases* 10: 222. https://doi.org/10.1186/1471-2334-10-222.

2. Bourouiba, L. (n.d.). Fluid and Health Network. Video gallery. https://lbourouiba.mit.edu/video-gallery.

3. Bourouiba, L., Dehandschoewercker, E., and Bush, J.W.M. (2014). Violent expiratory events: On coughing and sneezing. *Journal of Fluid Mechanics* 745: 537–563. https://doi.org/10.1017/jfm.2014.88.
4. Scharfman, B.E., et al. (2014). Visualization of sneeze ejecta: Steps of fluid fragmentation leading to respiratory droplets. *Experiments in Fluids* 57: 1–9.
5. Bourouiba chaired the 2019 Fluids and Health Conference, July 23 to August 2. https://fluids-health2019.mit.edu/.
6. Jones, N.R., et al. (2020). Two metres or one: What is the evidence for physical distancing in Covid-19? *BMJ* 370. https://doi.org/10.1136/bmj.m3223.
7. Bourouiba, L. (2021). The fluid dynamics of disease transmission. *Annual Review of Fluid Mechanics* 53: 473–508. https://doi.org/10.1146/annurev-fluid-060220-113712.
8. Hamner L., et al. (2020). High SARS-CoV-2 attack rate following exposure at a choir practice—Skagit County, Washington, March 2020. *MMWR* 69: 606–610. https://doi.org/10.15585/mmwr.mm6919e6.
9. COVID-19 Tracking Project. (n.d.). The Atlantic Monthly Group. https://covidtracking.com/data/national.
10. Gottlieb, S. (2021). *Uncontrolled Spread: Why COVID-19 Crushed Us and How We Can Defeat the Next Pandemic.* Harper Collins, New York.
11. Tang, J.W., et al. (2021). Covid-19 has redefined airborne transmission. *BMJ* 373. https://doi.org/10.1136/bmj.n913.
12. Riley, E.C., Murphy, G., and Riley, R.L. (1978). Airborne spread of measles in a suburban elementary school. *American Journal of Epidemiology* 107: 421–432. https://doi.org/10.1093/oxfordjournals.aje.a112560.
13. Word Health Organization. (2020, March 28). Tweet. https://twitter.com/who/status/1243972193169616898.
14. Slavitt, A. (2021). *Preventable: The Inside Story of How Leadership Failures, Politics, and Selfishness Doomed the U.S. Coronavirus Response.* St. Martin's Press, New York.
15. Lessler. J., et al. (2021). Household COVID-19 risk and in-person schooling. *Science* 372: 1092–1097. https://doi.org/10.1126/science.abh2939.
16. Prather, K.A., et al. (2020). Airborne transmission of SARS-CoV-2. *Science* 370: 303–304. https://doi.org/10.1126/science.abf0521.
17. Stetzenbach, L.D., Buttner, M. P., and Cruz, P. (2004). Detection and enumeration of airborne biocontaminants. *Current Opinion in Biotechnology* 15: 170–174. https://doi.org/10.1016/j.copbio.2004.04.009.
18. Morawska, L., and Cao, J. (2020). Airborne transmission of SARS-CoV-2: The world should face the reality. *Environment International* 139: 105730. https://doi.org/10.1016/j.envint.2020.105730.
19. Eisen, J. (2018). Applications being accepted for the 1st Microbiology of the Built Environment Gordon Research Conference. *microBEnet* (blog). https://microbe.net/2018/03/04/applications-being-accepted-for-the-1st-microbiology-of-the-built-environment-gordon-research-conference/.
20. Gordon Research Conference. (2018). Integrating human health with building microbiomes. Microbiology of the Built Environment, July15–20. https://www.grc.org/microbiology-of-the-built-environment-conference/2018/.

21. Virtual Issue Collection via Indoor Air (n.d.) *Indoor Air: Journal of the International Society of Indoor Air Quality and Climate.* https://onlinelibrary.wiley.com /journal/16000668.

22. ARPA-H. (n.d.). BREATHE: Building Resilient Environments for Air and Total Health. https://arpa-h.gov/research-and-funding/programs/breathe.

23. Allen, J.G., and Macomber, J.D. (2022). *Healthy Buildings: How Indoor Spaces Can Make You Sick—or Keep You Well.* 2nd ed. Harvard University Press, Cambridge, MA.

24. United States Environmental Protection Agency. (n.d.). Indoor air quality. https://www.epa.gov/report-environment/indoor-air-quality.

25. Leung, N.H.L., et al. (2020). Respiratory virus shedding in exhaled breath and efficacy of face masks. *Nature Medicine* 26: 676–680. https://doi.org/10.1038/s41591 -020-0843-2.

26. Eikenberry, S.E., et al. (2020). To mask or not to mask: Modeling the potential for face mask use by the general public to curtail the COVID-19 pandemic. *Infectious Disease Modelling* 5: 293–308. https://doi.org/10.1016/j.idm.2020.04.001.

27. Jarr, J. (2022, January 15). With COVID-19, air is both the problem and the solution. McGill Office for Science and Society. https://www.mcgill.ca/oss/article /covid-19/covid-19-air-both-problem-and-solution.

28. Emanuel, G. (2021, August 26). Does your kid's classroom need an air purifier? Here's how you can make one yourself. NPR. https://www.npr.org/sections/back -to-school-live-updates/2021/08/26/1031018250/does-your-kids-classroom-need -an-air-purifier-heres-how-you-can-make-one-yoursel.

29. See note 23.

30. CDC. (2021). CDC Scientific Brief: SARS-CoV-2 Transmission. https://archive.cdc .gov/#/details?url=https://www.cdc.gov/coronavirus/2019-ncov/science/science -briefs/sars-cov-2-transmission.html.

31. See note 14.

32. See note 2.

33. Morawska, L., and Milton, D.K. (2020). It is time to address airborne transmission of coronavirus disease 2019 (COVID-19). *Clinical Infectious Diseases* 71: 2311–2313. https://doi.org/10.1093/cid/ciaa939.

34. Allen, J. (2020, February 8). How health buildings can help us fight coronavirus. *Financial Times.* https://www.ft.com/content/5083fd42-4812-11ea-aee2-9ddb dc86190d.

35. See note 33.

36. Allen, J.G., and Marr, L.C. (2020, September 22). Yes, airborne transmission is happening. The CDC needs to set the record straight. *Washington Post.* https:// www.washingtonpost.com/opinions/2020/09/22/yes-airborne-transmission-is -happening-cdc-needs-set-record-straight/.

37. Prather, K.A., Wang, C.C., and Schooley, R.T. (2020). Reducing transmission of SARS-CoV-2. *Science* 368: 1422–1424. https://doi.org/10.1126/science.abc6197.

38. See note 33.

39. Wong, F., and Collins, J.J. (2020). Evidence that coronavirus superspreading is fat-tailed. *Proceedings of the National Academy of Sciences* 117: 29416–29418. https://doi.org/10.1073/pnas.2018490117.

40. See note 8.

41. CDC. (n.d.). *MMWR* Publications. https://www.cdc.gov/mmwr/publications /index.html.

42. Oran, D.P., and Topol, E.J. (2020). Prevalence of asymptomatic SARS-CoV-2 infection. *Annals of Internal Medicine*173: 362–367. https://doi.org/10.7326/M20-3012.

43. Prem, K., Cook, A.R., and Jit, M. (2017). Projecting social contact matrices in 152 countries using contact surveys and demographic data. *PLOS Computational Biology* 13: e1005697. https://doi.org/10.1371/journal.pcbi.1005697.

44. Feehan, D.M., and Mahmud, A.S. (2021). Quantifying population contact patterns in the United States during the COVID-19 pandemic. *Nature Communications* 12: 893. https://doi.org/10.1038/s41467-021-20990-2.

45. Poletti, P., et al. (2021). Association of age with likelihood of developing symptoms and critical disease among close contacts exposed to patients with confirmed SARS-CoV-2 infection in Italy. *JAMA Network Open* 4: e211085. https://doi.org /10.1001/jamanetworkopen.2021.1085.

46. Dowd, J.B., et al. (2020). Demographic science aids in understanding the spread and fatality rates of COVID-19. *Proceedings of the National Academy of Sciences*, 117: 9696–9698. https://doi.org/10.1073/pnas.2004911117.

47. Mossong, J., et al. (2008). Social contacts and mixing patterns relevant to the spread of infectious diseases. *PLOS Medicine* 5: e74. https://doi.org/10.1371/journal .pmed.0050074.

48. Odds are based on an independence assumption: the probability p that at least one individual in a group of size n (e.g., n = 25) is hospitalized when the risk of hospitalization is q (e.g., q = 0.002) is defined as $p = 1-(1-q)^n$.

49. Taquet, M., et al. (2022). Neurological and psychiatric risk trajectories after SARS-CoV-2 infection: an analysis of 2-year retrospective cohort studies including 1 284 437 patients. *The Lancet Psychiatry*, 9: 815–827. https://doi.org /10.1016/S2215-0366(22)00260-7.

50. Curiskis, A., et al. (2021, March 31). What we know—and what we don't know— about the impact of the pandemic on our most vulnerable community. *COVID-19 Tracking Project*. https://covidtracking.com/analysis-updates/what-we-know -about-the-impact-of-the-pandemic-on-our-most-vulnerable-community.

51. Karmakar, M., Lantz, P. M., and Tipirneni, R. (2021). Association of social and demographic factors with COVID-19 incidence and death rates in the US. *JAMA Network Open* 4: e2036462–e2036462. https://doi.org/10.1001/jamanetworkopen .2020.36462.

52. Mena, G.E., et al. (2021). Socioeconomic status determines COVID-19 incidence and related mortality in Santiago, Chile. *Science*, 372: eabg529. https://doi.org/10 .1126/science.abg5298.

53. Golodryga, B., and Pomrenze, Y. (2020, November 20). College students head home as coronavirus cases spike. CNN. https://www.cnn.com/2020/11/20/us /colleges-coronavirus-thanksgiving-break-wellness/index.html.

54. Dean, A., et al. (2022). Resident mortality and worker infection rates from COVID-19 lower in union than nonunion US nursing homes, 2020–21. *Health Affairs* 45: https://doi.org/10.1377/hlthaff.2021.01687.

55. Bagchi, S., et al. (2021). Rates of COVID-19 among residents and staff members in nursing homes—United States, May 25–November 22, 2020. *MMWR* 70: 52–55. https://doi.org/10.15585/mmwr.mm7002e2.

56. See notes 10 and 14.

57. Gostin, L.O., and Hodge, J.G., Jr. (2020). US emergency legal responses to novel coronavirus: balancing public health and civil liberties. *JAMA* 232: 1131–1132. https://doi.org/10.1001/jama.2020.2025.

58. World Health Organization. (2015). Ebola response roadmap situation report update, 14 January 2015. https://reliefweb.int/report/sierra-leone/ebola-response-roadmap-situation-report-update-14-january-2015.

59. WHO Ebola Response Team. (2014). Ebola virus disease in West Africa: the first 9 months of the epidemic and forward projections. *New England Journal of Medicine* 371: 1481–1495. https://pubmed.ncbi.nlm.nih.gov/25244186/.

60. Evans, D.K., Goldstein, M., and Popova, A. (2015). Health-care worker mortality and the legacy of the Ebola epidemic. *The Lancet Global Health*, 3: e439–e440. https://doi.org/10.1016/S2214-109X(15)00065-0.

61. Chowell, G., and Nishiura, H. (2014). Transmission dynamics and control of Ebola virus disease (EVD): a review. *BMC Medicine* 12. https://doi.org/10.1186/s12916-014-0196-0.

62. Donnelly, C.A., et al. (2003). Epidemiological determinants of spread of causal agent of severe acute respiratory syndrome in Hong Kong. *The Lancet* 361: 1761–1766. https://doi.org/10.1016/S0140-6736(03)13410-1.

63. Lau, J.T.F., et al. (2003). Monitoring community responses to the SARS epidemic in Hong Kong: from day 10 to day 62. *Journal of Epidemiology & Community Health* 57: 864–870. https://doi.org/10.1136/jech.57.11.864.

64. Anderson, R.M., et al. (2004). Epidemiology, transmission dynamics and control of SARS: the 2002–2003 epidemic. *Philosophical Transactions of the Royal Society of London, Series B: Biological Sciences* 359: 1091–1105. https://doi.org/10.1098/rstb.2004.1490.

65. Peiris, J.S.M., et al. (2003). Clinical progression and viral load in a community outbreak of coronavirus-associated SARS pneumonia: a prospective study. *The Lancet* 361: 1767–1772. https://doi.org/10.1016/S0140-6736(03)13412-5.

66. See note 64.

67. Du, Z., et al. (2020, March 20). The serial interval of COVID-19 from publicly reported confirmed cases. MedRxiv. https://doi.org/10.1101/2020.02.19.20025452. See the 2020 update in *Emerging Infectious Diseases* 26: 1341–1343. https://doi.org/10.3201/eid2606.200357.

Chapter 3. Asymptomatic Transmission Leads to Many More Fatalities

1. Nelson, E.J., et al. (2009). Cholera transmission: the host, pathogen and bacteriophage dynamic. *Nature Reviews Microbiology* 7: 693–702. https://doi.org/10.1038/nrmicro2204.

2. Gyles, C.L. (2007). Shiga toxin-producing *Escherichia coli*: an overview. *Journal of Animal Science*, 85 (S13): E45–E62. https://doi.org/10.2527/jas.2006-508.

3. Karimzadeh, S., Bhopal, R., and Nguyen Tien, H. (2021). Review of infective dose, routes of transmission and outcome of COVID-19 caused by the SARS-COV-2: comparison with other respiratory viruses. *Epidemiology & Infection* 149: E96. https://doi.org/10.1017/S0950268821000790.

4. Bar-On, Y.M., et al. (2020). SARS-CoV-2 (COVID-19) by the numbers. *eLife* 9: e57309. https://doi.org/10.7554/eLife.57309.

5. Sender, R., et al. (2021). The total number and mass of SARS-CoV-2 virions. *Proceedings of the National Academy of Sciences* 118: e2024815118. https://doi.org/10.1073/pnas.2024815118.

6. Wang, S., et al. (2020). Modeling the viral dynamics of SARS-CoV-2 infection. *Mathematical Biosciences* 328: 108438. https://doi.org/10.1016/j.mbs.2020.108438.

7. See note 5.

8. Zeng, C., et al. (2022). SARS-CoV-2 spreads through cell-to-cell transmission. *Proceedings of the National Academy of Sciences* 119: e2111400119. https://doi.org/10.1073/pnas.2111400119.

9. Gonçalves, A., et al. (2020). Timing of antiviral treatment initiation is critical to reduce SARS-CoV-2 viral load. *CPT: Pharmacometrics & Systems Pharmacology* 9: 509–514. https://doi.org/10.1002/psp4.12543.

10. Perelson, A.S., and Ke, R. (2021). Mechanistic modeling of SARS-CoV-2 and other infectious diseases and the effects of therapeutics. *Clinical Pharmacology & Therapeutics* 109: 829–840. https://doi.org/10.1002/cpt.2160.

11. Azkur, A.K., et al. (2020). Immune response to SARS-CoV-2 and mechanisms of immunopathological changes in COVID-19. *Allergy* 75: 1564–1581. https://doi.org/10.1111/all.14364.

12. McCormack, W., and Zimmer, C. (2020, June 26). Spit and "SWISH": Inside the NBA-Yale partnership aiming to validate a saliva-based test for COVID-19. *Yale Daily News*. https://yaledailynews.com/blog/2020/06/26/spit-and-swish-inside-the-nba-yale-partnership/.

13. Mateus, J., et al. (2020). Selective and cross-reactive SARS-CoV-2 T cell epitopes in unexposed humans. *Science* 370: 89–94. https://doi.org/10.1126/science.abd3871.

14. V'kovski, P., et al. (2021). Coronavirus biology and replication: implications for SARS-CoV-2. *Nature Reviews Microbiology* 19: 155–170. https://doi.org/10.1038/s41579-020-00468-6.

15. Li, Q., et al. (2020). Early transmission dynamics in Wuhan, China, of novel coronavirus–infected pneumonia. *New England Journal of Medicine* 382: 1199–1207. https://doi.org/10.1056/NEJMoa2001316.

16. Bedford, T., et al. (2020). Cryptic transmission of SARS-CoV-2 in Washington state. *Science* 370: 571–575. https://doi.org/10.1126/science.abc0523.

17. Deng, X., et al. (2020). Genomic surveillance reveals multiple introductions of SARS-CoV-2 into Northern California. *Science* 369: 582–587. https://doi.org/10.1126/science.abb9263.

18. Jijón, S., (2023). Using early detection data to estimate the date of emergence of an epidemic outbreak. MedRxiv. 2023.01.09.23284284. https://doi.org/10.1101/2023.01.09.23284284.

19. Fox-Lewis, A., et al. (2022). Airborne transmission of SARS-CoV-2 Delta variant within tightly monitored isolation facility, New Zealand (Aotearoa). *Emerging Infectious Diseases* 28: 501–509. https://doi.org/10.3201/eid2803.212318.

20. Wong, F., and Collins, J.J. (2020). Evidence that coronavirus superspreading is fat-tailed. *Proceedings of the National Academy of Sciences* 117: 29416–29418. https://doi.org/10.1073/pnas.2018490117.

21. Delamater, P.L., et al. (2019). Complexity of the basic reproduction number (R_0). *Emerging Infectious Diseases* 25: 1–4. https://doi.org/10.3201/eid2501.171901.

22. Anderson, R.M., and May, R.M. (1991). *Infectious Diseases of Humans: Dynamics and Control*. Oxford University Press, Oxford.

23. Diekmann, O., Heesterbeek, J.A.P., and Metz, J.A. (1990). On the definition and the computation of the basic reproduction ratio R_0 in models for infectious diseases in heterogeneous populations. *Journal of Mathematical Biology* 28: 365–382. https://doi.org/10.1007/BF00178324.

24. Kucharski, A. (2020) *The Rules of Contagion: Why Things Spread—and Why They Stop*. Basic Books, New York.

25. See note 24.

26. Liu, Y., Eggo, R.M., and Kucharski, A.J. (2020). Secondary attack rate and superspreading events for SARS-CoV-2. *The Lancet* 395: e47. https://doi.org/10.1016/S0140-6736(20)30462-1.

27. Park, S.W., et al. (2020). Reconciling early-outbreak estimates of the basic reproductive number and its uncertainty: framework and applications to the novel coronavirus (SARS-CoV-2) outbreak. *Journal of the Royal Society Interface* 17: 20200144. https://doi.org/10.1098/rsif.2020.0144.

28. Arino, J., et al. (2007). A final size relation for epidemic models. *Mathematical Biosciences and Engineering* 4: 159. https://doi.org/10.3934/mbe.2007.4.159.

29. See note 27.

30. Diamond, D. (2020, December 16). "We want them infected": Trump appointee demanded "herd immunity" strategy, emails reveal. Politico. https://www.politico.com/news/2020/12/16/trump-appointee-demanded-herd-immunity-strategy-446408.

31. Farrar, J. (2021). *Spike: The Virus vs. The People—the Inside Story*. Profile Books, London.

32. Bergmann, S., et al. (2020, July 21). Sweden hoped herd immunity would curb COVID-19. Don't do what we did. It's not working. *USA Today*. https://www.usatoday.com/story/opinion/2020/07/21/coronavirus-swedish-herd-immunity-drove-up-death-toll-column/5472100002/.

33. Editorial Board (2022, June 29). How one doctor wrecked the pandemic response. *Washington Post*. https://www.washingtonpost.com/opinions/2022/06/29/scott-atlas-covid-herd-immunity-strategy/.

34. Calmfors, L. (2022, October 20). We saved our economy in Sweden. But too many people died. *Washington Post*. https://www.washingtonpost.com/outlook/2020/10/20/sweden-economy-pandemic-strategy/.

35. Levitt, M. (2020, March 13). The Corona chronologies: part I. China. https://www.dropbox.com/s/am2437ywxnh4b84/CURRENT.Analysis_of_Coronavirus-2019_Data_Michael_Levitt.pdf?dl=0.

36. One prediction was that COVID-19 would be over in the United States by August 25, 2020. See Levitt, M. (2020, July 25). Tweet. https://twitter.com/MLevitt_NP2013/status/1287036738565738496?s=20&t=2Rex4ecZoBO5pCr5UNC73A.

37. Hébert-Dufresne, L., et al. (2020). Beyond R0: heterogeneity in secondary infections and probabilistic epidemic forecasting. *Journal of the Royal Society Interface* 17: 20200393. https://doi.org/10.1098/rsif.2020.0393.

38. Kissler, S.M., et al. (2020). Projecting the transmission dynamics of SARS-CoV-2 through the postpandemic period. *Science* 368: 860–868. https://doi.org/10.1126/science.abb5793.

39. Ferguson, N., et al. (2020, March 16). Report 9: Impact of non-pharmaceutical interventions (NPIs) to reduce COVID19 mortality and healthcare demand. Imperial College, London. https://doi.org/10.25561/77482.

40. Borrell, B. (2021). *The First Shots: The Epic Rivalries and Heroic Science Behind the Race to the Coronavirus Vaccine*. Mariner Books, New York.

41. Goldhill, O., et al. (2021, October 8). "Naively ambitious": How COVAX failed on its promise to vaccinate the world. Stat. https://www.statnews.com/2021/10/08/how-covax-failed-on-its-promise-to-vaccinate-the-world/.

42. Crook, H., et al. (2021) Long covid—mechanisms, risk factors, and management. *BMJ* 374: n1648. https://doi.org/10.1136/bmj.n1648.

43. Georgia DPH COVID-19 Status Report (2024, March 27). https://ga-covid19.ondemand.sas.com/.

44. COVID-19: Data. (n.d.). NYC Health. https://www.nyc.gov/site/doh/covid/covid-19-data-totals.page.

45. Russell, T.W., et al. (2020). Estimating the infection and case fatality ratio for coronavirus disease (COVID-19) using age-adjusted data from the outbreak on the Diamond Princess cruise ship, February 2020. *Eurosurveillance* 25: 2000256. https://doi.org/10.2807/1560-7917.ES.2020.25.12.2000256.

46. The COVID-19 Tracking Project. (n.d.). The Atlantic Monthly Group. https://covidtracking.com/data/national.

47. Najmabadi, S. (2020, June 27). Want a coronavirus test in Texas? You may have to wait for hours in a car. *Texas Tribune*. https://www.texastribune.org/2020/06/27/coronavirus-testing-texas/.

48. CDC. Estimated COVID-19 burden. https://archive.cdc.gov/#/details?url=https://www.cdc.gov/coronavirus/2019-ncov/cases-updates/burden.html.

49. Google. (2020–2022). COVID-19 community mobility reports. https://www.google.com/covid19/mobility.

50. State of New Jersey Governor's Office. (2020, April 8). Coronavirus updates and information: Governor Phil Murphy signs executive order. https://www.nj.gov/governor/news/news/562020/20200408e.shtml.

51. Kramer, S. (2020, August 27). More Americans say they are regularly wearing masks in stores and other businesses. *Pew Research Center.* https://www.pew research.org/fact-tank/2020/08/27/more-americans-say-they-are-regularly -wearing-masks-in-stores-and-other-businesses/.

52. Ballotpedia. (2022). State-level mask requirements in response to the coronavirus (COVID-19) pandemic, 2020–2022. https://ballotpedia.org/State-level_mask _requirements_in_response_to_the_coronavirus_(COVID-19)_pandemic, _2020-2022.

53. Fisher, K.A., et al. (2020). Factors associated with cloth face covering use among adults during the COVID-19 pandemic—United States, April and May 2020. *MMWR* 69: 933–937. https://doi.org/10.15585/mmwr.mm6928e3.

54. Peiris, J.S.M., et al. (2003). Coronavirus as a possible cause of severe acute respiratory syndrome. *The Lancet* 361: 1319–1325. https://doi.org/10.1016/S0140 -6736(03)13077-2.

55. Paules, C.I., Marston, H.D., and Fauci, A.S. (2020) Coronavirus infections—more than just the common cold. *JAMA* 323: 707–708. https://doi.org/10.1001/jama.2020 .0757.

56. Park, S.W., et al. (2023). Intermediate levels of asymptomatic transmission can lead to the highest epidemic fatalities. *PNAS Nexus* 2: pgad106. https://doi.org /10.1093/pnasnexus/pgad106.

57. Rohani, P., and Keeling, M. (2008) *Modeling Infectious Diseases in Humans and Animals.* Princeton University Press, Princeton, NJ.

Chapter 4. Respecting the Public

1. COVID-19 Tracking Project. (n.d.). The Atlantic Monthly Group. https://covid tracking.com/data/national.

2. Park, S.W., et al. (2020). The time scale of asymptomatic transmission affects estimates of epidemic potential in the COVID-19 outbreak. *Epidemics* 31, 100392. https://doi.org/10.1016/j.epidem.2020.100392.

3. This book focuses on events, reactions, and scientific discoveries that took place predominantly from 2020 to 2023, before Twitter became "X." The platform will be referred to as Twitter.

4. Lenski, R. (2017). Experimental evolution and the dynamics of adaptation and genome evolution in microbial populations. *The ISME Journal* 11: 2181–2194. https://doi.org/10.1038/ismej.2017.69.

5. Lenski, R. (2020, March 9). *Telliamed Revisited* (blog). https://telliamedrevisited .wordpress.com/2020/03/09/we-interrupt-this-experiment/.

6. Hadfield, J., et al. (2018). Nextstrain: real-time tracking of pathogen evolution. *Bioinformatics* 34: 4121–4123. https://academic.oup.com/bioinformatics/article /34/23/4121/5001388.

7. Neher, R. (2020, February 9). Tweet. https://twitter.com/richardneher/status /1226677060413751297?s=20&t=ujDnEkro7z95ZrBtwhYmTg.

8. Georgia Tech College of Sciences. (2020, February 11). Georgia Tech science forum spotlights coronavirus outbreak (news release). https://cos

.gatech.edu/news/georgia-tech-science-forum-spotlights-coronavirus
-outbreak.

9. Glim, M. (2021). A record-breaking sprint to create a COVID-19 vaccine. *NIH Intramural Blog.* https://irp.nih.gov/blog/post/2021/07/a-record-breaking-sprint
-to-create-a-covid-19-vaccine.

10. Cohen, J. (2020, January 11). Chinese researchers reveal draft genome of virus implicated in Wuhan pneumonia outbreak. *Science.* https://www.science.org
/content/article/chinese-researchers-reveal-draft-genome-virus-implicated
-wuhan-pneumonia-outbreak.

11. Zhang, Y-Z. (2020). Novel 2019 coronavirus genome SARS-CoV-2 coronavirus as communicated by Eddie Holmes via virological.org. https://virological.org/t/novel
-2019-coronavirus-genome/319.

12. Bedford, T. (2020, March 2). Cryptic transmission of novel coronavirus revealed by genomic epidemiology. *Bedford Lab* (blog). https://bedford.io/blog/ncov
-cryptic-transmission/.

13. Borrell, B. (2021). *The First Shots: The Epic Rivalries and Heroic Science Behind the Race to the Coronavirus Vaccine.* Mariner Books, New York.

14. Park, S.W., et al. (2020). Reconciling early-outbreak estimates of the basic reproductive number and its uncertainty: framework and applications to the novel coronavirus (SARS-CoV-2) outbreak. *Journal of the Royal Society Interface.* 17: 20200144. https://doi.org/10.1098/rsif.2020.0144.

15. Weitz, J.S. (2020). COVID-19 event risk assessment planner. Figshare. https://doi
.org/10.6084/m9.figshare.11965533.v1.

16. Weitz, J.S. (2020, March 10). Twitter. https://twitter.com/joshuasweitz/status
/1237556232304508928?s=20.

17. Arnold, C. (2020, March 26). COVID-19: Biomedical research in a world under social-distancing measures. *Nature Medicine.* https://www.nature.com/articles
/d41591-020-00005-1.

18. This risk estimator is equivalent to the binomial distribution, such that the estimated probability that at least one individuals is infected in a large group of size n can be approximated as $r = 100\% * [1-(1-p)^n]$ if the per capita probability of infection is p.

19. NCAA. (2020, March 12). NCAA cancels remaining winter and spring champion-ships. https://www.ncaa.org/news/2020/3/12/ncaa-cancels-remaining-winter-and
-spring-championships.aspx.

20. Gottlieb, S. (2021). *Uncontrolled Spread: Why COVID-19 Crushed Us and How We Can Defeat the Next Pandemic.* Harper, New York.

21. Lewis, M. (2021). *The Premonition: A Pandemic Story.* W.W. Norton, New York.

22. Slavitt, A. (2021). *Preventable: The Inside Story of How Leadership Failures, Politics, and Selfishness Doomed the U.S. Coronavirus Response.* St. Matin's Press, New York.

23. Mena Lora, A.J., et al. (2023). Rapid development of an integrated network infrastructure to conduct phase 3 COVID-19 vaccine trials. *JAMA Network Open* 6: e2251974. https://doi.org/10.1001/jamanetworkopen.2022.51974.

24. National Governors Association. (2020). Summary of public health criteria in reopening plans through June 9, 2020. https://www.nga.org/coronavirus-reopening-plans/.
25. Coglianese, C., and Mahboubi, N.A. (2021). Administrative law in a time of crisis: comparing national responses to COVID-19. *Administrative Law Review* 73: 1–19. https://administrativelawreview.org/wp-content/uploads/sites/2/2021/03/07.-ALR-73.1_Foreward_FINAL.pdf.
26. Sridhar, D. (2022). *Preventable: How a Pandemic Changed the World and How to Stop the Next One*. Penguin, Random House UK, London.
27. Farrar, J. (2021). *Spike: The Virus vs. The People—the Inside Story*. Profile Books, London.
28. Beckett, S.J., and Weitz, J.S. (2020, May 15). Georgia's reopening depended on missing data. *Slate*. https://slate.com/technology/2020/05/georgia-reopening-data-error.html.
29. Two prominent examples are the Johns Hopkins Coronavirus Resource Center (https://coronavirus.jhu.edu) and Our World in Data at Oxford (https://ourworldindata.org).
30. Andris, C. (2016). Integrating social network data into GISystems. *International Journal of Geographical Information Science* 30: 2009–2031. https://doi.org/10.1080/13658816.2016.1153103.
31. Weitz, J.S. (2020, July 7). Twitter. https://twitter.com/joshuasweitz/status/1280528852608077829?s=20.
32. Weitz, J. (2021, September 14). Communicating with 8 million people through Shiny. https://www.rstudio.com/speakers/joshua-weitz/.
33. Altmetric. (2020, November) Real-time, interactive website for US-county-level COVID-19 event risk assessment. https://nature.altmetric.com/details/93947263.
34. Eisenstein, M. (2021, January). What's your risk of catching COVID? These tools help you to find out. *Nature* 589: 158–159.
35. Sinclair, A.H., et al. (2021). Pairing facts with imagined consequences improves pandemic-related risk perception. *Proceedings of the National Academy of Sciences* 118: e2100970118. https://doi.org/10.1073/pnas.2100970118.
36. Sinclair, A.H., et al. (2021). Imagining a personalized scenario selectively increases perceived risk of viral transmission for older adults. *Nature Aging* 1: 677–683. https://doi.org/10.1038/s43587-021-00095-7.
37. Sinclair, A.H., et al. (2024). Scenario-based messages on social media motivate COVID-19 information seeking. *Journal of Applied Research in Memory and Cognition* 13: 124–135. https://doi.org/10.1037/mac0000114.
38. Allen, J.G., and Macomber, J.D. (2022). *Healthy Buildings: How Indoor Spaces Can Make You Sick—or Keep You Well*. 2nd ed. Harvard University Press, Cambridge, MA.
39. Bazant, M. Z., and Bush, J. W. (2021). A guideline to limit indoor airborne transmission of COVID-19. *Proceedings of the National Academy of Sciences* 118: e2018995118. https://doi.org/10.1073/pnas.2018995118.
40. Middleton, J., Reintjes, R., and Lopes, H. (2020). Meat plants—a new front line in the covid-19 pandemic. *BMJ* 370: m2716. https://doi.org/10.1136/bmj.m2716.

41. Ouslander, J.G., and Grabowski, D.C. (2020). COVID-19 in nursing homes: calming the perfect storm. *Journal of the American Geriatrics Society* 68: 2153–2162. https://doi.org/10.1111/jgs.16784.

42. Keeling, C.D., et al. (1976). Atmospheric carbon dioxide variations at Mauna Loa Observatory, Hawaii. *Tellus* 28: 538–551. https://doi.org/10.3402/tellusa.v28i6.11322.

43. Satish, U., et al. (2012). Is CO_2 an indoor pollutant? Direct effects of low-to-moderate CO_2 concentrations on human decision-making performance. *Environmental Health Perspectives* 120: 1671–1677. https://doi.org/10.1289/ehp.1104789.

44. Allen J.G., et al. (2016). Associations of cognitive function scores with carbon dioxide, ventilation, and volatile organic compound exposures in office workers: a controlled exposure study of green and conventional office environments. *Environmental Health Perspectives* 124: 805–812. https://doi.org/10.1289/ehp.1510037.

45. Mooney, C. (2021, February 10). The coronavirus is airborne. Here's how to know if you're breathing other people's breath. *Washington Post.* https://www.washingtonpost.com/health/2021/02/10/carbon-dioxide-device-coronavirus/.

46. Derk, R.C., et al. (2023). Efficacy of do-it-yourself air filtration units in reducing exposure to simulated respiratory aerosols. *Building and Environment* 229: 109920. https://doi.org/10.1016/j.buildenv.2022.109920.

47. Peng, Z., Miller, S.L., and Jimenez, J.L. (2023). Model evaluation of secondary chemistry due to disinfection of indoor air with germicidal ultraviolet lamps. *Environmental Science & Technology Letters* 10: 6–13. https://doi.org/10.1021/acs.estlett.2c00599.

48. Graeffe, F., et al. (2023). Unwanted indoor air quality effects from using ultraviolet C lamps for disinfection. *Environmental Science & Technology Letters* 10: 172–178. https://doi.org/10.1021/acs.estlett.2c00807.

49. Tang, C.S.K., and Wong, C.Y. (2004). Factors influencing the wearing of facemasks to prevent the severe acute respiratory syndrome among adult Chinese in Hong Kong. *Preventive Medicine* 39: 1187–1193. https://doi.org/10.1016/j.ypmed.2004.04.032.

50. Baxter-King, R. et al. (2022). How local partisan context conditions prosocial behaviors: Mask wearing during COVID-19. *Proceedings of the National Academy of Sciences USA: 119:* e2116311119. https://doi.org/10.1073/pnas.2116311119.

51. Cramer, M. (2021, January 26). Mask fights and a "mob mentality": what flight attendants faced over the last year. *New York Times.* https://www.nytimes.com/2021/01/26/business/airlines-capitol-violence.html.

52. Lu, J., et al. (2020). COVID-19 outbreak associated with air conditioning in restaurant, Guangzhou, China, 2020. *Emerging Infectious Diseases* 26: 1628–1631. https://doi.org/10.3201/eid2607.200764.

53. O'Sullivan, F. (2021, June 15). Paris will keep its Covid-era cafe terraces. *Bloomberg.* https://www.bloomberg.com/news/articles/2021-06-15/paris-will-keep-its-covid-era-cafe-terraces.

54. Gettings, J., et al. (2021). Mask use and ventilation improvements to reduce COVID-19 incidence in elementary schools—Georgia, November 16–December 11, 2020. *MMWR*, 70: 779. https://doi.org/10.15585/mmwr.mm7021e1.

55. Lyu, W., and Wehby, G. L. (2020). Community use of face masks and COVID-19: evidence from a natural experiment of state mandates in the US. *Health Affairs* 39: 1419–1425. https://doi.org/10.1377/hlthaff.2020.00818.

56. Howard, J., et al. (2021). An evidence review of face masks against COVID-19. *Proceedings of the National Academy of Sciences* 118: e2014564118. https://doi.org/10.1073/pnas.2014564118.

57. Jefferson T., et al. (2023). Physical interventions to interrupt or reduce the spread of respiratory viruses. *Cochrane Database of Systematic Reviews* 1: CD006207. https://doi.org/10.1002/14651858.CD006207.pub6.

58. Markowitz, A. (2020, July 20). State-by-state guide to face mask requirements. *AARP*. https://www.aarp.org/health/healthy-living/info-2020/states-mask-mandates-coronavirus.html. An updated version from January 25, 2022, was referenced.

59. Bokemper, S.E., et al. (2021). Experimental evidence that changing beliefs about mask efficacy and social norms increase mask wearing for COVID-19 risk reduction: results from the United States and Italy. *PLOS ONE* 16: e0258282. https://doi.org/10.1371/journal.pone.0258282.

60. Malecki, K.M.C., Keating, J.A., and Safdar, N. (2021). Crisis communication and public perception of COVID-19 risk in the era of social media. *Clinical Infectious Diseases* 72: 697–702. https://doi.org/10.1093/cid/ciaa758.

61. See note 28.

62. Bruine de Bruin, W., and Bennett, D. (2020). Relationships between initial COVID-19 risk perceptions and protective health behaviors: a national survey. *American Journal of Preventive Medicine* 59: 157–167. https://doi.org/10.1016/j.amepre.2020.05.001.

63. See note 33.

Chapter 5. Testing as a Form of Pandemic Mitigation

1. Rupar, A. (2020, May 15). Trump seems to think there'd be no coronavirus if there was no testing. It doesn't work like that. *Vox*. https://www.vox.com/2020/5/15/21259888/trump-coronavirus-testing-very-few-cases.

2. Granich, R.M., et al. (2009). Universal voluntary HIV testing with immediate antiretroviral therapy as a strategy for elimination of HIV transmission: a mathematical model. *The Lancet* 373: 48–57. https://doi.org/10.1016/S0140-6736(08)61697-9.

3. RECOVERY Collaborative Group. (2020). Effect of hydroxychloroquine in hospitalized patients with Covid-19. *New England Journal of Medicine* 383: 2030–2040. https://doi.org/10.1056/NEJMoa2022926.

4. Perrone, M., and Marchione, M. (2020, April 24). FDA warns of heart risks with Trump-promoted malaria drug. AP News. https://apnews.com/article/virus-outbreak-malaria-donald-trump-us-news-ap-top-news-21249a99b29d7b2c8648acb1f01a9812.

5. Temple, C., Hoang, R., and Hendrickson, R.G. (2021). Toxic effects from ivermectin use associated with prevention and treatment of Covid-19 (letter to the editor). *New England Journal of Medicine* 385: 2197–2198. https://doi.org/10.1056/NEJMc2114907.

6. Skipper, C.A., et al. (2020). Hydroxychloroquine in nonhospitalized adults with early COVID-19: a randomized trial. *Annals of Internal Medicine* 173: 623–631. https://doi.org/10.7326/M20-4207.

7. Shear, M.D., and Haberman, M. (2020, April 22). Health Dept. official says doubts on hydroxychloroquine led to his ouster. *New York Times.* https://www.nytimes.com/2020/04/22/us/politics/rick-bright-trump-hydroxychloroquine-coronavirus.html.

8. CDC. (2021, August 24). Coronavirus disease 2019 (COVID-19): 2021 case definition. https://ndc.services.cdc.gov/case-definitions/coronavirus-disease-2019-2021.

9. Boyce N. (2020). Bills of Mortality: tracking disease in early modern London. *The Lancet.* 395: 1186–1187. https://doi.org/10.1016/S0140-6736(20)30725-X.

10. Karlinsky, A., and Kobak, D. (2021). Tracking excess mortality across countries during the COVID-19 pandemic with the World Mortality Dataset. *eLife* 10: e69336. https://doi.org/10.7554/eLife.69336.

11. These figures are from the Johns Hopkins University Coronavirus Resource Center (https://coronavirus.jhu.edu/region/united-states), which collected US data until March 10, 2023.

12. Keeling, M.J., Hollingsworth, T.D., and Read, J.M. (2020). Efficacy of contact tracing for the containment of the 2019 novel coronavirus (COVID-19). *Journal of Epidemiology and Community Health* 74: 861–866. https://doi.org/10.1136/jech-2020-214051.

13. Kurnai, N., et al. (2021). COVID-19 test prices and payment policy. *Peterson-KFF Health System Tracker.* https://www.healthsystemtracker.org/brief/covid-19-test-prices-and-payment-policy.

14. University of Illinois System. (n.d.). UIUC SHIELD-based PCR testing platform: overview. https://www.iasb.com/IASB/media/General/IDPH-SHIELD-IL-overview-051021.pdf.

15. Chinazzi, M., et al. (2020). The effect of travel restrictions on the spread of the 2019 novel coronavirus (COVID-19) outbreak. *Science* 368: 395–400. https://doi.org/10.1126/science.aba9757.

16. Colizza, V., et al. (2006). The role of the airline transportation network in the prediction and predictability of global epidemics. *Proceedings of the National Academy of Sciences* 103: 2015–2020. https://doi.org/10.1073/pnas.0510525103.

17. Lee, J.S., et al. (2021). Analysis of the initial lot of the CDC 2019-Novel Coronavirus (2019-nCoV) real-time RT-PCR diagnostic panel. *PLOS ONE* 16: e0260487. https://doi.org/10.1371/journal.pone.0260487.

18. Cohen, J. (2020). The United States badly bungled coronavirus testing—but things may soon improve. *Science.* https://doi.org/10.1126/science.abb5152.

19. Gottlieb, S. (2020, February 2). Tweet. https://twitter.com/ScottGottliebMD/status/1224044448193171459?s=20.

20. Gottlieb, S. (2021). *Uncontrolled Spread: Why COVID-19 Crushed Us and How We Can Defeat the Next Pandemic.* Harper, New York.

21. See note 20—reporting synthesis was already available by February 28, 2020.
22. Mina, M.J., and Andersen, K.G. (2021). COVID-19 testing: One size does not fit all. *Science* 371: 126–127. https://doi.org/10.1126/science.abe9187.
23. Tirrell, M., Wells, N. and Miller, L. (2020, August 15). Forty percent of US Covid-19 tests come back too late to be clinically meaningful, data show. CNBC. https://www.cnbc.com/2020/08/15/forty-percent-of-us-covid-19-tests-come-back-too-late-to-be-clinically-meaningful-data-show.html.
24. Wymant, C., et al. (2021). The epidemiological impact of the NHS COVID-19 app. *Nature* 594: 408–412. https://doi.org/10.1038/s41586-021-03606-z.
25. Mathieu, E., et al. (2022). Coronavirus (COVID-19) testing. *Our World in Data*. https://ourworldindata.org/coronavirus-testing.
26. Jegerlehner, S., et al. (2021). Diagnostic accuracy of a SARS-CoV-2 rapid antigen test in real-life clinical settings. *International Journal of Infectious Diseases* 109: 118–122. https://doi.org/10.1016/j.ijid.2021.07.010.
27. Gibson, G., et al. (2021). Surveillance-to-diagnostic testing program for asymptomatic SARS-CoV-2 infections on a large, urban campus in fall 2020. *Epidemiology* 33: 209–216. https://doi.org/10.1097/EDE.0000000000001448.
28. Ranoa, D.R.E., et al. (2022). Mitigation of SARS-CoV-2 transmission at a large public university. *Nature Communications* 13: 3207. https://doi.org/10.1038/s41467-022-30833-3.
29. Denny, T.N., et al. (2020). Implementation of a pooled surveillance testing program for asymptomatic SARS-CoV-2 infections on a college campus—Duke University, Durham, North Carolina, August 2–October 11, 2020. *MMWR* 69: 1743. https://doi.org/10.15585/mmwr.mm6946e1.
30. Paltiel, A.D., Zheng, A., and Walensky, R.P. (2020). Assessment of SARS-CoV-2 screening strategies to permit the safe reopening of college campuses in the United States. *JAMA Network Open* 3: e2016818–e2016818. https://doi.org/10.1001/jamanetworkopen.2020.16818.
31. Larremore, D.B., et al. (2021). Test sensitivity is secondary to frequency and turnaround time for COVID-19 screening. *Science Advances* 7: eabd5393. https://doi.org/10.1126/sciadv.abd5393.
32. Gibson, G., and Weitz, J.S. (2020, August 4). Science and projects for a return to campus. Georgia Institute of Technology. https://figshare.com/articles/presentation/Science_and_Projections_for_a_Return_to_Campus/12761357.
33. See note 28.
34. Stirgus, E. (2020, July 6). University System of Georgia to require masks in classrooms after all. *Atlanta Journal Constitution*. https://www.ajc.com/news/local-education/university-system-georgia-require-masks-classrooms-after-all/VyTlGue4hfyynzl2snRHqK/.
35. R1 universities are those in the top tier in terms of research activity according to the Carnegie Classification of Institutions of Higher Education (https://carnegieclassifications.acenet.edu/classification_descriptions/basic.php).
36. Mutesa, L., et al. (2021). A pooled testing strategy for identifying SARS-CoV-2 at low prevalence. *Nature* 589: 276–280. https://doi.org/10.1038/s41586-020-2885-5.

37. Gelman, A., and Carpenter, B. (2020). Bayesian analysis of tests with unknown specificity and sensitivity. *Applied Statistics* 69: 1269–1283. https://doi.org/10.1111/rssc.12435.

38. CMS. (n.d.). Clinical Laboratory Improvement Amendments (CLIA). https://www.cms.gov/regulations-and-guidance/legislation/clia

39. See note 32.

40. Georgia Tech. (2020). Twitter. August 26, 2020. https://twitter.com/GeorgiaTech/status/1298685524132200448?s=20.

41. CDC Community Level. (Updated 2024, February 20). https://data.cdc.gov/Public-Health-Surveillance/Weekly-COVID-19-County-Level-of-Community-Transmis/jgk8-6dpn/about_data.

42. Christie, A., et al. (2021). Guidance for implementing COVID-19 prevention strategies in the context of varying community transmission levels and vaccination coverage. *MMWR* 70: 1044–1047. https://doi.org/10.15585/mmwr.mm7030e2.

43. Spokane City Council. (2021, December 13). 2022 adopted budget. https://static.spokanecity.org/documents/budget/2022/2022-adopted-budget.pdf.

44. Spiers, J. (2022, March 6). Mayor Stoney presents Richmond's $836M general fund budget for FY23. *Richmond BizSense*. https://richmondbizsense.com/2022/03/06/mayor-stoney-presents-richmonds-836m-general-fund-budget-for-fy23/.

45. Havers, F.P., et al. (2020). Seroprevalence of antibodies to SARS-CoV-2 in 10 sites in the United States, March 23–May 12, 2020. *JAMA Internal Medicine* 180: 1576–1586. https://doi.org/10.1001/jamainternmed.2020.4130.

46. McLaughlin, K. (2021, December 7). Growing use of home Covid-19 tests leaves health agencies in the dark about unreported cases. Stat. https://www.statnews.com/2021/12/07/growing-use-of-home-covid19-tests-leaves-health-agencies-in-the-dark/.

47. University of Oxford. (2023, March). COVID-19 infection survey. https://www.ndm.ox.ac.uk/covid-19/covid-19-infection-survey.

48. Polo, D., et al. (2020). Making waves: Wastewater-based epidemiology for COVID-19–approaches and challenges for surveillance and prediction. *Water Research* 186: 116404. https://doi.org/10.1016/j.watres.2020.116404.

49. Weidhaas, J., et al. (2021). Correlation of SARS-CoV-2 RNA in wastewater with COVID-19 disease burden in sewersheds. *Science of the Total Environment* 775: 145790. https://doi.org/10.1016/j.scitotenv.2021.145790.

50. Karthikeyan, S., et al. (2021). Rapid, large-scale wastewater surveillance and automated reporting system enable early detection of nearly 85% of COVID-19 cases on a university campus. *mSystems* 6: e00793-21. https://doi.org/10.1128/mSystems.00793-21.

51. Smyth, D.S., et al. (2022). Tracking cryptic SARS-CoV-2 lineages detected in NYC wastewater. *Nature Communications* 13: 635. https://doi.org/10.1038/s41467-022-28246-3.

52. Johansson, M.A., et al. (2021). SARS-CoV-2 transmission from people without COVID-19 symptoms. *JAMA Network Open* 4: e2035057–e2035057. https://doi.org/10.1001/jamanetworkopen.2020.35057.

53. Phillips, S., and Williams, M.A. (2021). Confronting our next national health disaster—long-haul Covid. *New England Journal of Medicine* 385: 577–579. https://doi.org/10.1056/NEJMp2109285.

54. Ochieng, N., et al. (2021, January 14). Factors associated with COVID-19 cases and deaths in long-term care facilities: findings from a literature review. *KFF*. https://www.kff.org/coronavirus-covid-19/issue-brief/factors-associated-with-covid-19-cases-and-deaths-in-long-term-care-facilities-findings-from-a-literature-review/.

55. Kahn, R., et al. (2022). Mathematical modeling to inform vaccination strategies and testing approaches for coronavirus disease 2019 (COVID-19) in nursing homes. *Clinical Infectious Diseases* 74: 597–603. https://doi.org/10.1093/cid/ciab517.

56. New York Times. (2021, June 1). Nearly one-third of US coronavirus deaths are linked to nursing homes. https://www.nytimes.com/interactive/2020/us/coronavirus-nursing-homes.html.

57. Consulat Général de France à Washington. (2022). Health pass: what to know if you are traveling to France. https://washington.consulfrance.org/health-pass-what-to-know-if-you-are-traveling-to-france.

58. Guedj, L., and Woo, Y. (2021, July 31). Thousands protests against COVID-19 health pass in France. Reuters. https://www.reuters.com/world/europe/thousands-protest-against-covid-19-health-pass-france-2021-07-31/.

59. Borrell, B. (2021). *The First Shots: The Epic Rivalries and Heroic Science Behind the Race to the Coronavirus Vaccine.* Mariner Books, New York.

Chapter 6. Vaccination Requires More than Vaccines

1. Dearlove, B., et al. (2020). A SARS-CoV-2 vaccine candidate would likely match all currently circulating variants. *PNAS* 117: 23652–23662. https://doi.org/10.1073/pnas.2008281117.

2. Pardi, N., et al. (2018). mRNA vaccines—a new era in vaccinology. *Nature Reviews Drug Discovery* 17: 261–279. https://doi.org/10.1038/nrd.2017.243.

3. Mena Lora, A.J., et al. (2023). Rapid development of an integrated network infrastructure to conduct phase 3 COVID-19 vaccine trials. *JAMA Network Open.* 6: e2251974. https://doi.org/10.1001/jamanetworkopen.2022.51974.

4. Holder, J. (2023). Tracking coronavirus vaccinations around the world. *New York Times.* https://www.nytimes.com/interactive/2021/world/covid-vaccinations-tracker.html.

5. Polack, F.P., et al. (2020). Safety and efficacy of the BNT162b2 mRNA Covid-19 vaccine. *New England Journal of Medicine* 383: 2603–2615. https://doi.org/10.1056/NEJMoa2034577.

6. These percentages are from Our World in Data and its international COVID-19 dataset (https://ourworldindata.org/covid-vaccinations).

7. Pulliam, J.R., et al. (2022). Increased risk of SARS-CoV-2 reinfection associated with emergence of Omicron in South Africa. *Science* 376: eabn4947. https://doi.org/10.1126/science.abn4947.

8. CDC Data Tracker. (2023). COVID-19 vaccinations in the United States. https://covid.cdc.gov/covid-data-tracker/#vaccinations_vacc-total-admin-rate-total.

9. CDC. (2023). Trends in demographic characteristics of people receiving COVID-19 vaccinations in the United States. https://covid.cdc.gov/covid-data -tracker/#vaccination-demographics-trends.

10. Wolf, C. (2022). COVID vaccination rates vary in Trump vs. Biden counties. *US News.* https://www.usnews.com/news/health-news/articles/2022-01-27/counties -that-voted-for-trump-have-lower-covid-vaccination-rates.

11. See notes 6 and 8.

12. CDC. (2022, September 13). United States confirmed as country with circulating vaccine-derived poliovirus (news release). https://www.cdc.gov/media/releases /2022/s0913-polio.html#:~:text=Circulating%20vaccine-derived%20poliovirus %20occurs,in%20the%20oral%20polio%20vaccine.

13. Hill, H.A, et al. (2023). Vaccination coverage by age 24 months among children born during 2018–2019: National Immunization Survey–child, United States, 2019–2021. *MMWR* 72: 33–38. https://doi.org/10.15585/mmwr.mm7202a3.

14. Kirzinger, A., et al. (2021, November 16). KFF COVID-19 Vaccine Monitor: the increasing importance of partisanship in predicting COVID-19 vaccination status. *KFF.* https://www.kff.org/coronavirus-covid-19/poll-finding/importance -of-partisanship-predicting-vaccination-status.

15. Wright, A. (2021, April 23). Republican men are vaccine-hesitant, but there's little focus on them. *Stateline.* https://www.pewtrusts.org/en/research-and-analysis /blogs/stateline/2021/04/23/republican-men-are-vaccine-hesitant-but-theres-little -focus-on-them.

16. Siegler, A.J., et al. (2021). Trajectory of COVID-19 vaccine hesitancy over time and association of initial vaccine hesitancy with subsequent vaccination. *JAMA Network Open* 4: e2126882. https://doi.org/10.1001/jamanetworkopen.2021.26882.

17. Karlamangle, S. (2022). Once Known for Vaccine Skeptics, Marin Now Tells Them 'You're Not Welcome'. *New York Times.* October 2, 2022. https://www .nytimes.com/2022/10/02/us/covid-vaccine-marin-california.html

18. Godlee, F., Smith, J., and Marcovitch, H. (2011). Wakefield's article linking MMR vaccine and autism was fraudulent. *BMJ* 342: c7452. https://doi.org/10.1136/bmj .c7452.

19. Mara, J. (2015, January 31). California measles outbreak highlights Marin vaccination dilemma. *Marin Independent Journal.* https://www.marinij.com/2015 /01/31/california-measles-outbreak-highlights-marin-vaccination-dilemma/.

20. Allday, E. (2019, March 1). Measles outbreak in Bay Area in 2018 tied to unvacci- nated children. *San Francisco Chronicle.* https://www.sfchronicle.com/health /article/Measles-outbreak-in-Bay-Area-in-2018-tied-to-13656990.php.

21. County of Marin. (2019, June 5). Child vaccinations (news release). https://www .marincounty.org/main/county-press-releases/press-releases/2019/hhs -vaccinations-060519.

22. Bauch, C.T., and Earn, D.J. (2004). Vaccination and the theory of games. *Proceedings of the National Academy of Sciences* 101: 13391–13394. https://doi.org/10.1073/pnas .0403823101.

23. Hardin, G. (1968). The tragedy of the commons. *Science* 162: 1243–1248. https://doi .org/10.1126/science.162.3859.1243.

24. Weitz, J.S., et al. (2016). An oscillating tragedy of the commons in replicator dynamics with game-environment feedback. *Proceedings of the National Academy of Sciences* 113: E7518–E7525. https://doi.org/10.1073/pnas.1604096113.
25. Kates, J., Tolbert, J., and Rouw, A. (2022, January 19). The red/blue divide in COVID-19 vaccination rates continues: an update. *KFF*. https://www.kff.org/policy-watch/the-red-blue-divide-in-covid-19-vaccination-rates-continues-an-update/.
26. Johnson, A.G., et al. (2022). COVID-19 incidence and death rates among unvaccinated and fully vaccinated adults with and without booster doses during periods of Delta and Omicron variant emergence—25 US jurisdictions, April 4–December 25, 2021. *MMWR* 71:132–138. http://dx.doi.org/10.15585/mmwr.mm7104e2.
27. Johnson, A.G., et al. (2023). COVID-19 incidence and mortality among unvaccinated and vaccinated persons aged ≥12 years by receipt of bivalent booster doses and time since vaccination—24 US jurisdictions, October 3, 2021–December 24, 2022. *MMWR* 72: 145–152. https://doi.org/10.15585/mmwr.mm7206a3.
28. Wells, C.R., and Galvani, A.P. (2022). The global impact of disproportionate vaccination coverage on COVID-19 mortality. *The Lancet Infectious Diseases* 22: 1254–1255. https://doi.org/10.1016/S1473-3099(22)00417-0.
29. Lance, R. (2021, June 29). How COVID-19 vaccines were made so quickly without cutting corners. *Science News*. https://www.sciencenews.org/article/covid-coronavirus-vaccine-development-speed.
30. Kolata, G., and Mueller, B. (2022, January 15). Halting progress and happy accidents: how mRNA vaccines were made. *New York Times*. https://www.nytimes.com/2022/01/15/health/mrna-vaccine.html.
31. Gupta, S., and Loberg, K. (2021). *World War C: Lessons from the Covid-19 Pandemic and How to Prepare for the Next One.* Simon & Schuster, New York.
32. Borrell, B. (2021). *The First Shots: The Epic Rivalries and Heroic Science Behind the Race to the Coronavirus Vaccine.* Mariner Books, New York.
33. Wrapp, D., et al. (2020). Cryo-EM structure of the 2019-nCoV spike in the prefusion conformation. *Science* 367: 1260–1263. https://doi.org/10.1126/science.abb2507.
34. Shioda, K., et al. (2021). Estimating the cumulative incidence of SARS-CoV-2 infection and the infection fatality ratio in light of waning antibodies. *Epidemiology* 32: 518. https://doi.org/10.1097/EDE.0000000000001361.
35. Cao, Y., et al. (2022). Omicron escapes the majority of existing SARS-CoV-2 neutralizing antibodies. *Nature* 602: 657–663. https://doi.org/10.1038/s41586-021-04385-3.
36. Cohen, J. (2017, September 20). Why flu vaccines so often fail. *Science*. https://doi.org/10.1126/science.aaq0105.
37. Booker, B. (2020, December 15). Fauci predicts U.S. could see signs of herd immunity by late March or early April. NPR. https://www.npr.org/sections/coronavirus-live-updates/2020/12/15/946714505/fauci-predicts-u-s-could-see-signs-of-herd-immunity-by-late-march-or-early-april.
38. See note 8.

39. Brooks Harper, K. (2021, March 9). Texans don't have to prove they're eligible for the COVID-19 vaccine and some are jumping the line. Here's why. *Texas Tribune*. https://www.khou.com/article/news/health/coronavirus/vaccine/texans-vaccine-line-skipping-1a-1b-no-proof-they-are-eligible/285-cb64809a-c978-47f9-b131-076b1c180d04.

40. Thompson, S.A. (2020, December 3). Find your place in the vaccine line. *New York Times*. https://www.nytimes.com/interactive/2020/12/03/opinion/covid-19-vaccine-timeline.html.

41. Gupta, S. (2020, March 24). Is it ever OK to skip the vaccine line? We asked an expert. CNN. https://www.cnn.com/2021/03/24/health/coronavirus-vaccine-line-jumping-ethics-gupta-wellness/index.html.

42. Numbers cited are from the COVID-19 Data Explore archives of the Our World in Data dataset from Oxford University (https://ourworldindata.org/covid-cases).

43. Crotty, S. (2021). Hybrid immunity. *Science* 372: 1392–1393. https://doi.org/10.1126/science.abj225.

44. Hui, D.S. (2021). Hybrid immunity and strategies for COVID-19 vaccination. *The Lancet Infectious Diseases* 23: 2–3. https://doi.org/10.1016/S1473-3099(22)00640-5.

45. Figures cited are from the CDC's COVID Data Tracker (https://covid.cdc.gov/covid-data-tracker).

46. Barnes, O., et al. (2022, March 14). Hong Kong Omicron deaths expose limits of fraying zero-Covid policy. *Financial Times*. https://www.ft.com/content/6e610cac-400b-4843-a07b-7d870e8635a3.

47. Figures on coronavirus (COVID-19) deaths are from Our World in Data, Oxford University (https://ourworldindata.org/covid-deaths).

48. Bubar, K.M., et al. (2021). Model-informed COVID-19 vaccine prioritization strategies by age and serostatus. *Science* 371: 916–921. https://doi.org/10.1126/science.abe6959.

49. De Kruif, P. (2002). *Microbe Hunters*. Harcourt, San Diego, CA.

50. Amin, K., et al. (2022, April 21). COVID-19 mortality preventable by vaccines. *Peterson-KFF Health System Tracker*. https://www.healthsystemtracker.org/brief/covid19-and-other-leading-causes-of-death-in-the-us/.

51. Watson, O.J., et al. (2022). Global impact of the first year of COVID-19 vaccination: a mathematical modelling study. *The Lancet Infectious Diseases* 22:1293–1302. https://doi.org/10.1016/S1473-3099(22)00320-6.

52. Yamey, G., et al. (2022). It is not too late to achieve global Covid-19 vaccine equity. *BMJ* 376: e070650. https://doi.org/10.1136/bmj-2022-070650.

53. Thompson, H.S., et al. (2021). Factors associated with racial/ethnic group–based medical mistrust and perspectives on COVID-19 vaccine trial participation and vaccine uptake in the US. *JAMA Network Open* 4: e2111629. https://doi.org/10.1001/jamanetworkopen.2021.11629.

54. Reiter, P.H. (2020). Acceptability of a COVID-19 vaccine among adults in the United States: How many people would get vaccinated? *Vaccine* 38: 6500–6507. https://doi.org/10.1016/j.vaccine.2020.08.043.

55. Kirzinger, A., et al. (2021, November 16). KFF COVID-19 Vaccine Monitor: the increasing importance of partisanship in predicting COVID-19 vaccination status. *KFF*. https://www.kff.org/coronavirus-covid-19/poll-finding/importance -of-partisanship-predicting-vaccination-status/.

56. Sinclair, A.H., et al. (2023). Reasons for receiving or not receiving bivalent COVID-19 booster vaccinations among adults—United States, November 1–December 10, 2022. *MMWR* 72: 73–75. https://doi.org/10.15585/mmwr.mm7203a5.

57. See note 56.

58. Ebinger, J.E., et al. (2021). Antibody responses to the BNT162b2 mRNA vaccine in individuals previously infected with SARS-CoV-2. *Nature Medicine* 27: 981–984. https://doi.org/10.1038/s41591-021-01325-6.

59. Keen, A. (2021, March 19). Harriet A. Washington on the narrative around vaccine hesitancy in the African American community. *Keen On* (podcast). https://lithub .com/harriet-a-washington-on-the-narrative-around-vaccine-hesitancy-in-the -african-american-community/.

60. Thomas, S.B., and Quinn, S.C. (1991). The Tuskegee Syphilis Study, 1932 to 1972: implications for HIV education and AIDS risk education programs in the black community. *American Journal of Public Health* 81: 1498–1505. https://doi.org /10.2105/AJPH.81.11.1498.

61. Christensen, J. (2021). In rural Georgia, a door-to-door push to get neighbors vaccinated against Covid-19. CNN. July 13, 2021. https://www.cnn.com/2021/06 /06/health/rural-vaccination-randolph-county-georgia/index.html.

62. Ivory, D., Leatherby, L., and Gebeloff, R. (2021, April 17). Least vaccinated US counties have something in common: Trump voters. *New York Times*. https:// www.nytimes.com/interactive/2021/04/17/us/vaccine-hesitancy-politics.html.

63. Ouldali, N., et al. (2022). Hyper inflammatory syndrome following COVID-19 mRNA vaccine in children: a national post-authorization pharmacovigilance study. *The Lancet Regional Health–Europe* 17: 100393. https://doi.org/10.1016/j .lanepe.2022.100393.

64. Sparks, G., et al. (2022). KFF COVID-19 Vaccine Monitor: pregnancy misinformation—May 2022. *KFF*. https://www.kff.org/coronavirus-covid-19/poll -finding/kff-covid-19-vaccine-monitor-pregnancy-misinformation-may-2022/.

65. CDC. (2013, September 12). Selected adverse events reported after COVID-19 vaccination. https://www.cdc.gov/coronavirus/2019-ncov/vaccines/safety/adverse -events.html.

66. CDC. (2022, September 6). Diphtheria, tetanus, and whooping cough vaccination. https://www.cdc.gov/vaccines/vpd/dtap-tdap-td/public/index.html.

67. American College Health Association. (n.d.). Vaccines and immunizations. https://www.acha.org/ACHA/Resources/Topics/Vaccine.aspx.

68. Bar-On, Y.M., et al., (2021). Protection of BNT162b2 vaccine booster against Covid-19 in Israel. *New England Journal of Medicine* 385: 1393–1400. https://doi.org /10.1056/NEJMoa2114255.

69. CDC. Resource page for vaccines for COVID-19. https://www.cdc.gov/coronavirus /2019-ncov/vaccines/index.html.

70. Bar-On, Y.M., et al. (2022). Protection by a fourth dose of BNT162b2 against Omicron in Israel. *New England Journal of Medicine* 386: 1712–1720. https://doi.org/10.1056/NEJMoa2201570.

71. Kim, J.H., Marks, F., and Clemens, J.D. (2021). Looking beyond COVID-19 vaccine phase 3 trials. *Nature Medicine* 27: 205–211. https://doi.org/10.1038/s41591-021-01230-y.

72. See note 33.

73. Du, L., et al. (2009). The spike protein of SARS-CoV—a target for vaccine and therapeutic development. *Nature Reviews Microbiology* 7: 226–236. https://doi.org/10.1038/nrmicro2090.

74. Hotez, P.J. (2023). SARS-CoV-2 variants offer a second chance to fix vaccine inequities. *Nature Reviews Microbiology* 21, 127–128. https://doi.org/10.1038/s41579-022-00824-8.

75. Havers, F.P., et al. (2020). Seroprevalence of antibodies to SARS-CoV-2 in 10 sites in the United States, March 23–May 12, 2020. *JAMA Internal Medicine* 180: 1576–1586. https://doi.org/10.1001/jamainternmed.2020.4130.

76. CDC. Archived webpage for estimated COVID-19 burden. https://archive.cdc.gov/www_cdc_gov/coronavirus/2019-ncov/cases-updates/burden.html.

77. Larremore, D.B., et al. (2021). Estimating SARS-CoV-2 seroprevalence and epidemiological parameters with uncertainty from serological surveys. *eLife* 10: e64206. https://doi.org/10.7554/eLife.64206.

78. Weitz, J.S., et al. (2020). Modeling shield immunity to reduce COVID-19 epidemic spread. *Nature Medicine* 26: 849–854. https://doi.org/10.1038/s41591-020-0895-3.

79. Norheim, O.F. (2020). Protecting the population with immune individuals. *Nature Medicine* 26: 823–824. https://doi.org/10.1038/s41591-020-0896-2.

80. Kraay, A.N.M., et al. (2021). Modeling serological testing to inform relaxation of social distancing for COVID-19 control. *Nature Communications* 12: 7063. https://doi.org/10.1038/s41467-021-26774-y.

81. CDC. (2024, April 25). Nationwide COVID-19 infection-induced antibody seroprevalence (commercial laboratories). https://covid.cdc.gov/covid-data-tracker/#national-lab.

82. Jecker, N.S., Wightman, A. G., and Diekema, D. S. (2021). Vaccine ethics: an ethical framework for global distribution of COVID-19 vaccines. *Journal of Medical Ethics* 47: 308–317. https://doi.org/10.1136/medethics-2020-107036.

83. Moodley K. (2022). Vaccine inequity is unethical. *Nature Human Behaviour* 6: 168–169. https://www.nature.com/articles/s41562-022-01295-w.

84. Stiglitz, J.E. (2022). Vaccinating the world against COVID-19 is a no-brainer. *PLOS Global Public Health* 2: e0000427. https://doi.org/10.1371/journal.pgph.0000427.

85. Shivam, S., Weitz, J.S., and Wardi, Y. (2022). Vaccine stockpile sharing for selfish objectives. *PLOS Global Public Health* 2: e0001312. https://doi.org/10.1371/journal.pgph.0001312.

Coda

1. Pieper, K.J, Tang, M., and Edwards, M.A. (2017) Flint water crisis caused by interrupted corrosion control: investigating "ground zero" home. *Environmental Science and Technology* 51: 2007–2014. https://doi.org/10.1021/acs.est .6b04034.

2. Felton, E., and Pietsch, B. (2022, August 30). Jackson's water crisis comes after years of neglect: "We've been going it alone." *Washington Post*. https:// www.washingtonpost.com/nation/2022/08/30/jackson-mississippi-water-crisis -update/.

3. Hauser, C. (2023, March 3). How the Ohio train derailment and its aftermath unfolded. *New York Times*. https://www.nytimes.com/article/ohio-train-derailment -timeline.html.

4. Albarracín, D., et al. (2022). *Getting to and Sustaining the Next Normal: A Roadmap for Living with COVID*. Rockefeller Foundation, New York. https://www.rockefeller foundation.org/wp-content/uploads/2022/03/Getting-to-and-Sustaining-the-Next -Normal-A-Roadmap-for-Living-with-Covid-Report-Final.pdf.

5. Christakis, N. (2020). *Apollo's Arrow: The Profound and Enduring Impact of Coronavirus on the Way We Live*. Little Brown, New York.

6. CDC. (2022). Whooping cough is deadly for babies. https://www.cdc.gov/pertussis /pregnant/mom/deadly-disease-for-baby.html.

7. Barry, J.M. (2005) *The Great Influenza: The Story of the Deadliest Pandemic in History*. Penguin Books, New York.

Note: Page numbers followed by *f* or *t* indicate a figure or table asymptomatic transmission: averaging over age groups, 100; chain of, 210; comparative transmission potential, 94; context-related risk factors, 124–125; description, 65–67, 124; increased fatalities from, 92–95, 92*f*, 93*f*; mix with symptomatic transmission, 209–210; shedding of virus, 68, 69*f*; size of respiratory droplets, 66; stages of transmission, 68; strategies for reducing transmission, 125–134; symptomatic frequency comparison, 25, 36, 92; time/distance risk factors, 65–66; virus shedding and, 21, 65, 71–72, 210. *See also* transmission/transmissibility

at-home work, 70

Atlas, Scott, 18

avoidance strategies: distancing interventions, 6, 39–40, 43, 45, 86, 154; flu *vs.* COVID-19, 34; ignoring of precautions, 14; influence of socioeconomic status, 32; mask mandates, 34, 87, 88*f*, 129, 131, 137; pandemic, first year, 31–32; quarantining, 17, 60–61, 72, 99, 151*f*, 161. *See also* isolation of individuals; lockdowns

Bedford, Trevor, 101, 102

behavior change: asymptomatic transmission and, 91*t*; challenges in modifying, 123; influence of mandates, 86–87; making decisions about, 123; risk factors, 123; risk misestimation and, 122*t*; Sinclair's work on, 117–118, 118*t*, 122*t*; types of, 86

Bendavid, Eran, 23. *See also* Santa Clara Serological Survey

Bhattacharya, Jay, 23–24. *See also* Santa Clara Serological Survey

Biden, Joseph, 172

bioaerosols, 46

Biomedical Advanced Research and Development Agency, 136–137

Blacks, vaccination rates, 172

boosters (vaccination boosters), 189, 199–202; discovering people in need of, 203; mRNA, primary/second bivalent boosters, 171–172, 196, 200; in New Zealand, for older people, 189; political affiliation and, 172; role in risk reduction, 200–201

Bourouiba, Lydia, 37–38, 38*f*, 42, 46

Bright, Rick, 136–137

case ascertainment, 15–16

case fatality rate (CFR), 60, 84–86, 90

Centers for Disease Control and Prevention (CDC): adoption of holistic metric of community spread, 160–161; communication infrastructure, 110; early stance on, 40, 41; initial communication inadequacy, 110; survey on mask use, 87; 2020–2022, COVID-19 *vs.* flu deaths data, 28, 29*t*; 2021, update on airborne spread, 46

Centers for Medicare and Medicaid Services, 18

Chande, Aroon, 114

children: deaths by age group, 30, 31*t*, 32*t*, 33; deaths from flu *vs.* COVID, 29, 29*t*; mild/asymptomatic infections, 58; possible effects of variants, 34; risks in school settings, 50

China. *See* Guangzhou, China, long-distance transmission; Wuhan Province of China

Clinical Laboratory Improvement Amendments (CLIA), testing protocol, 156–157

colleges and universities, 53–56; age-related similarities, 53; comparison with long-term care facility, 52–53; fraternity house example, 53–55; isolation of students, 155, 158; next-day viral testing, 57; outbreak in dorms, 52; testing/intervention initiatives, 95, 152–159, 153*f*; variances in testing/intervention programs, 154–155

communication: initial CDC/WHO inadequacies, 110; need for geographic variances, 113; political/partisan-related challenges, 110–111; response strategies and, 59; risk models and, 105–109; tools for building platforms for, 109–117. *See also* COVID-19 Event Risk Assessment Planning Tool

communities: age-specific mixing, 53; benefit of mask wearing, 130–133; benefit of vaccines, 176; impact of disavowal of airborne transmission, 41, 46–47; perception of severity in, 54; population-level transmission, 9; risk control in, 165–169; role of testing at scale, 139, 152; spread of infection in susceptible populations, 176–177, 177f; wastewater testing in, 164. *See also* colleges and universities; long-term care (LTC) facilities; nursing homes; Skagit Valley Chorale super-spreading event; Wuhan Province of China

COVID-19 Event Risk Assessment Planning Tool (Georgia Tech): cognitive neuroscience interventions analysis, 117–118, 119, 120, 121f, 122f, 123; description, 104f; development/release of, 113, 117; interest as a research website, 132–133; use of an ascertainment bias, 115f; use to compare estimates, 117–118

cross-immunity, 71

cubic model (Hassett), 13–14

deaths/death rates. *See* fatalities/fatality rates

Delta wave, 180, 186, 188, 195f

Diamond Princess cruise ship, infection/fatality study, 17–18, 99

Dushoff, Jonathan, 101

Ebola virus disease (EVD), 59–60, 72, 74, 165

Environmental Protection Agency (EPA), 43

epidemic dynamics: with asymptomatic infections, 90t; description, 77–78; idealized spread over multiple generations, 89t; with symptomatic/infected individuals, 91t; synthetic simulation of, 78, 79f

epidemics, decline of. *See* susceptible depletion process

error function (erf) model, 9–12, 14

exponential growth, 67, 67f, 75–76, 78

exposed/incubation period, 20

Facebook, 24

false negatives, 27, 149

false positives, 26–28, 143–144, 156, 162

Farr, William, 10, 78. *See also* Farr's law of epidemics

Farr's law of epidemics: description, 10–11; Hassett's cubic model comparison, 13–14; use of, in AIDS study, 11–12, 12f

fatalities/fatality rates: adults, by age group, 31t, 32t, 33; adults, from COVID

vs. flu, 29t, 32t, 33; case fatality rate (CFR), 60, 84–86, 90; children, by age group, 30, 31t, 32t, 33; children, from flu *vs.* COVID, 29, 29t; COVID-19 *vs.* the flu, 28–38; *Diamond Princess* study findings, 17–18, 99; first pandemic year death data, 56, 130; first wave misestimation, 15–20; IHME zero death prediction, 4; impact of vaccinations, 171; infection fatality rate (IFR), 85–86, 163; linked to asymptomatic transmission, 92–95, 92f, 93f; Lombardy region, Italy, 15–16, 24, 51t, 72, 99; in long-term care (LTC) facilities, 58; preventability of, 180; SARS-1 *vs.* SARS-2 rates, 60; seasonal flu *vs.* COVID-19, 19; Skagit Valley superspreading event, 39–43, 47–48; 2020–2022, influenza *vs.* COVID-19, 28–29, 29t, 32; 2021, in Georgia/New York City, 84; 2021, US data, 180–181, 189; U.S., estimate of excess deaths, 139f

"A Fiasco in the Making? As the Coronavirus Pandemic Takes Hold, We Are Making Decisions without Reliable Data" (Ioannidis), 16–17

first wave: IHME Director's comments on, 4; misestimation of fatality rates, 15–20

forecasts/forecasting, 5f, 6–7; by IHME, 5f, 6–7, 9; role of accurate estimates of cases, 137

Gates Foundation, 3

Georgia Tech. *See* COVID-19 Event Risk Assessment Planning Tool; March Madness event

Guangzhou, China, long-distance transmission, 47–48, 49f

Hadfield, James, 101

Hanage, Bill, 4

handwashing, 37, 42

Harvard T.H. Chan School of Public Health, 4

Hassett, Kevin, 13–14

herd immunity: description, 76, 77f, 78–79, 178; rationale for pushing for, 81; role of population-based vaccination campaigns, 82; threshold of, 78–80, 80f, 178–179; vaccine-derived, 184

Hilley, Troy, 114

Hispanics, vaccination rates, 172
HIV (human immunodeficiency virus), 11, 135, 197
Hodcroft, Emma, 101
Hoover Institute, Stanford University, 18
hospitalization: age-specific risks for, 29, 32, 32*t*, 55; of children, 34; impact of two-dose mRNA vaccine, 198; for influenza, 36–37; in the intensive care unit, 5*f*, 15, 50, 85; limited likelihood for college students, 52; of long-term care residents, 52, 55–56; pandemic fatigue and, 134; population immunity and, 191; role of boosters in avoiding, 199, 201; SARS-1 *vs.* SARS-2, 60; SARS-1 *vs.* SARS-2 rates, 60; severity metrics, 83–84; timeline for, 7; underreporting and, 9
hybrid immunity, 188, 191

ICU (intensive care unit), 5*f*, 15, 50, 85
IHME. *See* Institute of Health Metrics and Evaluation
immunity: cross-immunity, 71; hybrid immunity, 188, 191; infection-derived, 176, 178, 192, 195; population-level, 81, 178, 187–188, 190*f*, 191–196, 195*f*; vaccine-derived, 170, 178, 184, 188. *See also* herd immunity
infection-derived immunity, 176, 178, 192, 195
infection fatality rate (IFR), 85–86, 163
influenza *vs.* COVID-19, fatality rates, 28–38; age 75+, 29, 29*t*; children (ages 1–14), 29, 29*t*; heart disease/cancer comparison, 31; newborns/infants, 29, 29*t*; older age groups, 29, 29*t*, 30, 31*t*, 32*t*, 33; 2020–2022, demographic comparison, 28–29, 29*t*, 32
Institute for Health Metrics and Evaluation (IHME) model: error function (erf) basis of early predictive forecasts, 9–12, 14; goal/mission of, 3–4; national/global predictions, 4, 5*f*; original model 4–6, 5*f*, 4, 5*f*; type of data, 4; zero deaths predictions, 3–4, 12
intensive care units (ICUs), 5*f*, 15, 50
Ioannidis, John, 16–20, 22–25; article on frequency of research findings, 25–26; diagnosis/testing recommendations, 19–20; fatality assumptions made by, 19;

range of potential outcomes for fatality rates, 18; STAT news website opinion piece, 16–17, 19
isolation of individuals, 20, 34, 70; by asymptomatic individuals, 140; barriers/challenges, 140–141; effectiveness of, 60–61, 144; between living quarters, 54; post-symptom isolation, 147; reasons for, 87, 91, 92*f*; of secondary cases, 141*f*, 150–151; of students at colleges, 155, 158; symptom-based, 93*f*; time determination, 107, 142*f*, 151*f*; use of testing and, 151, 161
Italy: cohort study results, 52; Lombardy region fatalities, 15–16, 24, 51*t*, 72, 99; Milan region lockdowns, 15

Johnson & Johnson, 171, 181
Journal of the American Medical Association, 11

Kilpatrick, Mark, 27

Lee, Seohla, 114
Lenski, Richard, 100–101
lockdowns: debates *versus* opening up, 124; impact of, 34; individual reactions to, 13; influence on behavior change, 86; Milan, Italy region, 15; reasons for, 137; stay-at-home orders, 3, 40, 99, 104
Lombardy region, Italy, 15–16, 24, 51*t*, 72, 99
long-term care (LTC) facilities, 56–58; age-related similarities, 53; comparison with college dorm, 52–53; first pandemic year fatalities data, 130; infection severity, hospitalizations, death, 58; mask wearing strategy for visitors, 130; need for tiered systems for airborne risk, 211; outbreaks in, 52; potential for impact of testing at, 211; staff member infections, 57–58; timing of outbreaks, 57; visitation risk factors, 166. *See also* nursing homes

March Madness event, 104*f*, 108–109
Marin County, vaccine hesitancy, 179–181
Marr, Linsey, 43, 46
masks/mask mandates: age-related use, 87; CDC survey on use of, 87; challenges in getting compliance, 133; effectiveness of, 65; enforcement decision, 129–130; Georgia school district study, 131;

incorrect/intermittent use of, 131–132; for long-term care facilities, 130; reasons for, 137; statewide mandates, 87, 88f; for targeted settings, 133; 2020 usage data, 87; types of, 44

mechanistic models, 6–7

MedRxiv, electronic sharing mechanism, 61

Meyers, Lauren Ancel, 61

Milton, Donald, 44, 46

MMR vaccine (measles, mumps, rubella), 176

Moderna mRNA vaccine, 170, 181

Morawska, Lidia, 44, 46

Morbidity and Mortality Weekly Report (MMWR) (CDC), 47

mRNA vaccines: comparative effectiveness chart, 182f; global distribution differences, 171–174; Moderna vaccine, 170, 181; Pfizer-BioNTech BNT162b2 vaccine, 172, 181, 182f; primary/second bivalent boosters, 171–172, 196, 200; rapid development of, 9, 102; speed, safety, efficacy of, 170–171, 192–193; updating for future viruses, 199–202

Murray, Chris, 3–4. *See also* IHME

N95 quality masks, 44

nasal swab samples, 21, 22, 148, 155

National Academy of Sciences, 100

National Institutes of Health (NIH), 171

Neal, Keith, 4

Neher, Richard, 101

Nextstrain, open-source toolkit, 101

non-Hispanic whites, vaccination rates, 172

nursing homes: first pandemic year deaths data, 56, 130; mask wearing strategy for visitors, 130; need for tiered systems for airborne risk, 211; potential for impact of testing at, 165; staff member infections, 57–58. *See also* long-term care (LTC) facilities

Omicron wave, 119, 168, 180, 189, 195f

Operation Warp Speed, 111

pandemic fatigue, 134

Park, Sang Woo, 101

Pfizer-BioNTech BNT162b2 mRNA vaccine, 172, 181, 182f

PLOS Medicine, 25

population-level immunity, 81, 178, 187–188, 190f, 191–196

population-scale vulnerability, 71

population-wide immune surveys, 202–205

Portugal, vaccine distribution rate, 171

Prather, Kimberly, 43, 46

public health campaigns, 55, 117, 209

quarantining, 17, 60–61, 72, 99, 151f, 161. *See also* isolation of individuals

recovery: chronic post-recovery challenges, 84; for college students, 55; herd immunity and, 178; long COVID, 84; testing rate and, 151–152, 151f

reverse transcription polymerase chain reaction (RT-PCR) tests: comparison to at-home antigen tests, 85; identification of SARS-CoV-2, 47–48; mechanisms of, 20–23, 22f, 143; use in finding infections, 68–70, 69f; viral RNA shedding result, 148

Rishishwar, Lavanya, 114

risk models: calculation analogy, 107–108; communication and, 105–109, 133; map-based estimate of risk, 114–116, 118, 119, 121f; principles of, 108; risk maps, 114, 116–117, 133; risk nowcasting/forecasting, 9, 132–134, 137; transmission events and, 105–106; transmission risk reports, 134; value of assessment tools, 133. *See also* COVID-19 Event Risk Assessment Planning Tool

risks/risk factors: for adults (60+/70+), 50–51, 51t; of asymptomatic transmission, 124–125; benefits of learning about, 123; of changing behavior, 123; for children, in school settings, 50; control in vulnerable communities, 165–169; for exposure/transmission at events, 107–109; gender-related data, 51t; misestimation of, 122t; prevaccination fatality risk assessment, 84; time and distance, 65–66

saliva samples, 21–23, 148, 155, 158

Santa Clara Serological Survey, 23–28; comparison to Lombardy region findings, 24; description, 23–24; false positives, 26–28; findings/influence of findings, 25; pushback/critique of scientific preprint of findings, 26–28

Santangelo, Phil, 101–102

SARS-1 outbreak, 60, 91, 128, 200; epidemiological impacts of, 60–61; mask wearing in response to, 128; SARS-CoV-2 comparison, 60–61, 63

SARS-CoV-2: concepts of epidemiological models, 72–74; "exposed"/"incubation" period, 20; first identification/genome sequencing, 170; hypotheses on observed *vs.* expected cases, 7–9; particles to initiate an infection, 65; positive test on *Diamond Princess* cruise ship, 17; RT-PCR tests identification of, 47–48; SARS-1 comparison, 60–61, 63; serial interval measure, 61–63, 62*t*; transmission at different sized events, 109; 2020, documented US cases, 106; viral testing for, 20–23; virus particle size, 45, 66

Schooley, Robert, 46

schools: reopening of, 34; risk of transmission, 50. *See also* colleges and universities

serial interval measure: defined, 61; negative values, 62–63, 62*f*; in SARS-CoV-2, 61–63, 62*t*

serological surveys, 24, 26, 142*f*, 156, 202–203. *See also* Santa Clara Serological Survey

severity: hospitalization metrics, 83–84; long-term care (LTC) facilities, 58; outbreak metrics, 83–84; symptoms, transmission, and, 59–63

Silver, Nate, 12–13

Sinclair, Allie, 117–118, 120*f*, 122*f*

single-ply masks, 44

Skagit Valley Chorale superspreading event, 39–43; COVID infections, deaths, 40; influence of singing on air dispersal, 39–40; lessons learned from, 47; parsimonious explanation for, 48

smallpox outbreaks, 10

sneezes, 36–38, 38*f*, 42–43, 70

soccer matches and transmission (Italy), 15

social media: communication of scientists on, 100, 103; influence on individual perceptions, 133; influencer-driven anti-vaccine sentiment, 197; map-based estimate of risk on, 114, 120*f*; release of quantitative estimates on, 109. *See also* Twitter

social/physical-distancing interventions, 6, 39–40, 43, 45, 86, 154

South Africa, vaccine distribution rate, 171

Spain, vaccine distribution rate, 171

stay-at-home orders, 3, 40, 99, 104

Strategic National Stockpile (of masks), 42

superspreader events: conditions for, 108; parsimonious explanation for (airborne spread), 48; Skagit Valley Chorale event, 39–43, 47, 48; strategy for reducing frequency, size, 123, 126, 208

susceptible depletion process, 76–77, 77*f*, 81

symptomatic infection: asymptomatic frequency comparison, 25, 36, 92; boosters and, 201; in college students, 54, 151; comparative transmission potential, 94; diagnosis of, 86; epidemic dynamics, 89*t*, 90*t*, 91*t*; healthy air landscape and, 125; link with age, 32, 50–51, 51*t*, 56; NBA players example, 69*f*; in nursing homes, 58; pneumonia-like symptoms, 40; potential signs of, 70; protective role of vaccines, 181–183, 182*f*; rapid spread of, 52; reliability of, 19; role of symptom recognition, 147; self-awareness of having, 87–88; severity of, 56, 59–63; superspreader event causative for, 103; timing of onset, 7, 20; transmissibility of, 37, 39, 46, 48, 56, 59–63; use of symptom-based behavior change, 87–88, 91, 91*t*, 95, 151; variability of, 8–9, 20, 68

testing, 135–169; access issues, 85–86; amount/frequency determination, 148; backlogs in results, 86; benefits of early testing, 140; benefits of testing close contacts, 141*f*; CLIA testing protocol, 156–157; college/university initiatives, 95, 152–159; consequences of late results, 141–142; delay between testing and receipt of results, 145*f*; disease status *vs.* transmission impact, 142*f*; drive-through centers, 86–86; early inadequacies, 8–9; environment-based, 162; false negatives, 27, 149; false positives, 26–28, 143–144, 156, 162; impact of limited capacity for, 16–17; impact on individual spread of days since infection, 149*f*; infection time determination, 150–151, 151*f*; Ioannidis's recommendations for antibody surveys, 19–20, 22–23; Italian cohort study, 52; as a means of mitigation, 137–138; mitigation potential of, 139–147; nasal swab samples, 21, 22, 148, 155; next-day viral testing, 57; public health goals addressed by, 136; rapid testing, 22, 95, 130, 162; rate relative to infectious period, 151–152; reasons for, 135, 137–138, 140, 147–148, 159; regional variances, 85; role in preventing more cases, 159–165; saliva samples, 21–23, 148, 155, 158; Santa Clara study, 26; scaling up strategies, 147–152; sensitivity, specificity, and, 148–151; serological assay kit, 24; for signs of viral presence and past, 20–23; state-level apps, 146; testing surveys, 162; Trump's comment on, 135; 2020, viral tests data, 146; undertesting/underreporting issues, 7, 30, 104–105; variances in college testing/interventions, 154–155; voluntary testing, 162–163; wastewater surveillance, 162, 164–165. *See also* reverse transcription polymerase chain reaction (RT-PCR) tests

transmission/transmissibility: associated modes of, 37; average duration of infectiousness, 73; basic reproduction number, 73; Bedford's warning on, 102; decreases in case counts, 75–83; of Ebola virus, 60; epidemiological models, 73–75; exponential growth of infection, 73–75, 75*f*; factors, 71; herd immunity and, 78–83, 80*f*; and increases in case counts, 71–75; in indoor environments, 43; long-distance infection example, 47–48, 49*f*; risk factors, 105–106; Skagit Valley Chorale example, 39–41, 47; speed of population-level transmission, 9; susceptible depletion process, 76–77, 77*f*, 81; symptoms, severity, and, 59–63; time/distance factors, 65–66; U.S. *vs.* Wuhan Province, 8, 15; viral load's link with, 61–62; virus requirements for, 72. *See also* airborne spread (transmission); asymptomatic transmission

Trump, Donald, 13, 135; comment on testing, 136; hydroxychloroquine recommendation, 136; vaccination rates during presidency, 172

tweets (on Twitter): by Neher, 101; by Silver, 13; by Weitz, 103, 104*f*, 108; by WHO, 41

Twitter, 100, 103, 108, 111

UEFA Championship League (soccer), 15
UV light, 44

vaccines/vaccination, 170–205; administration at scale, home, abroad, 196–199; benefits for communities, 176; benefits for non-vaccinated people, 178; benefits of, 81–82; Blacks/Hispanics, rates, 137; consequences of not being vaccinated, 14; conservative *vs.* liberal dichotomies, 172, 179; declining levels of people getting, 185; disparities, 172–173, 173*f*; efficacy variance, 184; failures to vaccinate, 185–192; getting the most benefit from, 193; global variances in distribution, 171–174; goal of public health officials, 178–179; herd immunity and, 81; hesitation about, 192; impact on measles in the U.S., 174–176m175*f*; infection reduction rates, 171; level of protection of, 183–184; Marin County, vaccine hesitancy, 179–181; mechanics of curbing epidemic spread, 174–179; misinformation about, 192; MMR vaccine, 176; Pfizer mRNA clinical trials, 181–182, 182*f*; political identity and, 172; possible post-vaccine infection, 182–183; potential trajectories of campaigns, 190*f*; prevaccination fatality risk assessment, 84; rapid development of, 9, 82–83; rates of Blacks/Hispanics/non-Hispanic whites, 172; reasons for, 137; scale of, in the U.S., 170; scaling up of delivery, 171; skeptics' anti-vaccine narrative, 186–192; social media anti-vaccine sentiment, 197; spread of infection in susceptible population, 176–177, 177*f*; state vaccination rates, 172–173, 173*f*; success of Operation Warp Speed, 111; symptoms in the unvaccinated, 54; 2022, differences in US rates, 173*f*; unvaccinated rate, 172; U.S., introduction of childhood vaccines, 176; vaccine-derived population immunity, 170, 178, 184, 188. *See also* boosters variants: ability to escape detection, 184, 194; CDC infrastructure and, 203; continuous evolution of, 207; current landscape of, 195f; Delta wave, 180, 186, 188, 195f; impact on children, 34; infections of vaccinated individuals, 108; Omicron wave, 119, 168, 180, 189, 195f; rapid, unexpected emergence, 200; wastewater systems and, 105

ventilation: asymptomatic transmission and, 124, 128, 210; importance of, 126–127; improvements in, 95, 114, 116–117; information on websites, 114; low-cost approaches, 116–117; paths for the redesign of, 127; risks of poor ventilation, 124, 128; role in stopping indoor spread, 44–45; ventilation rates, 45; wearing masks and, 129–130

ventilator use in hospitals, 4, 5f, 201

Verma, Seema, 18

viral load: detectability challenges, 20–21; increasing load signs, 21; link to transmissibility, 61–62; low viral load, 20; in NBA players (example), 69f, 70; peak levels for SARS-1, 60; schematic of relationships, 22f

viral RNA, 20–21, 23, 143, 148, 164

viral tests (reverse transcription polymerase chain reaction tests): increasing viral load signs, 21; mechanisms of, 20–21; timing of positivity, 21, 22f

virus shedding: asymptomatic transmission, 21, 65, 71–72, 210; PCR test evidence of, 148; positive antigen tests evidence of, 22

Wang, Chia, 46

wastewater surveillance, 162, 164–165

websites: map-based estimate of risk, 114–116, 118, 119, 121f; Nextstrain, 101; risk misestimation/behavior change, 122f; STAT news site, 16; vaccination location information, 196–197. *See also* COVID-19 Event Risk Assessment Planning Tool

working from home, 31

World Health Organization (WHO), 37; consequences of disavowal of airborne spread, 41–42; downplaying of airborne transmission, 40; initial communication inadequacy, 110; updated information on airborne spread, 46

Wuhan Province of China: age-related fatality data, 18; first case of SARS-CoV-2, 71; infection fatality rate, 7, 15, 99; long-distance transmission example, 47–48; 2020 report from, 99; U.S. comparison with, 8

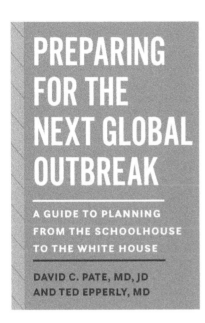
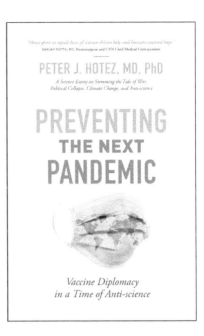
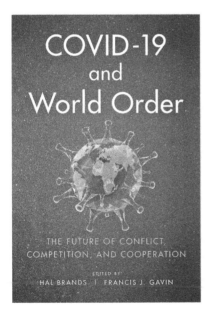
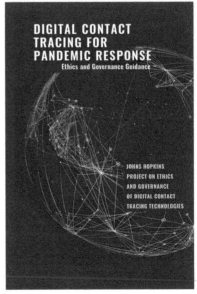

Milton Keynes UK
Ingram Content Group UK Ltd.
UKHW040812080924
447993UK00001B/1